Up to LOSE 10 POUNDS in 2 WEEKS

Dedicated to the millions of people
who are committed to losing weight.
May you live a happy and healthy life.

By Alex A. Lluch, Health & Fitness Expert
Author of Over 3 Million Books Sold!

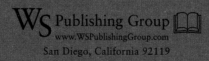

WS Publishing Group
www.WSPublishingGroup.com
San Diego, California 92119

Lose Up to 10 Pounds in 2 Weeks

By Alex A. Lluch

Nutritional and fitness guidelines based on information provided by the United States Food and Drug Administration, Food and Nutrition Information Center, National Agricultural Library, Agricultural Research Service, and the U.S. Department of Agriculture.

For more best-selling titles by WS Publishing Group,
visit www.wspublishinggroup.com

Image Credits:
Food icons: iStockphoto/stdemi (seafood)
Food icons: iStockphoto/Jane Norton (condiments)
Food icons: iStockphoto/Viviyan (fast foods, coffee, cupcakes)
Food icons: iStockphoto/Kristina Smirnova (alcoholic beverages)
Food icons: iStockphoto/RoccoMontoya (jam)
Food icons: iStockphoto/DimensionsDesigns (taco)

Exercise photos:
Tawn Tu, www.knightphotovideo.com
Aaron Tsai, www.aaroneye.com

ISBN 978-1-936061-17-4

Printed in China

contents

contents

Introduction

You know the frightening statistics by now: Sixty-seven percent of Americans are overweight, with 34 percent being considered obese. Millions of people are struggling with their weight every day and suffering the effects, from lack of energy to infertility to diabetes to heart disease. Perhaps most tangible, however, are the feelings of frustration, disappointment and self-doubt that trying to lose weight and failing bring. And many times, the last 10 pounds are the most difficult and stressful to lose. You may have already lost a great deal of weight but are struggling with a particularly stubborn 10 pounds. Or, you may be very close to your ideal weight, but having a hard time jumpstarting your metabolism or getting the motivation to lose the extra 10 pounds.

That's because so many diets are doomed to fail. They either force you to go cold turkey with the foods you love (causing cravings and bingeing), tell you to substitute real food with an unappealing powdered drink or meal replacement bar, or promote fast and easy weight loss through eating only certain foods and eliminating whole food groups (read: the lemonade-and-cayenne pepper diet or the grapefruit diet; extremely unhealthy). None of these types of diets are healthy or sustainable, meaning you'll only gain the weight right back afterward. And you're not learning any new eating or exercise habits, so you'll simply revert back to your old lifestyle, the one that made you gain weight in the first place.

The *Lose Up to 10 Pounds in 2 Weeks* diet and fitness program, however, is full of the most powerful, proven secrets in the world to help you lose the weight you want in record time. Slim down for a class reunion, vacation, birthday celebration, or just because swimsuit season is never far off. Or maybe there's no special occasion; maybe you're just tired of carrying around 10 or more extra pounds and you know, with a little dedication and several fast lifestyle changes, you can be at weight you want. Being healthier, happier and in better shape with more energy are always the best reasons for losing weight. Medical research has shown that losing just 5 to 10 percent of your body weight can significantly improve a person's health by lowering cholesterol and the risk of heart disease, stroke and diabetes.

What's interesting about this program is that the amount of weight you're trying to lose is a deceptive amount — it's not 100 pounds, it's about 10. Seems like it should be easy, right? Well, of course it's not. Someone who needs to lose 100 pounds burns many more calories just by going through his or her day with all that extra weight. But someone who is slimmer, who wants to lose just a few pounds, is burning far fewer calories than a heavier person. Consider running on a treadmill for an hour — when you start, the machine requires you to enter your weight. That is because an hour of running at the same intensity burns many fewer calories for someone who is 150 pounds, than for someone who is 200 pounds. Additionally, as we age and our metabolisms slow down, the body gets comfortable with the extra pounds and it's tougher to lose them. Your body needs a jumpstart, just like a car with a stalled battery! You'll find the diet and fitness tips in this book to be just what you need to get moving more efficiently, cooking smarter, planning ahead, and eating better. And unlike other diets, where you're eliminating the nutrients your body truly needs, you won't be starving or exhausted. This program is what is considered a "flexible diet," one that instructs dieters to monitor the consumption of calories to lose weight. You won't starve, eat only one kind of food or miss out on dinners with friends or your favorite treats — you just need to implement the diet and fitness secrets you'll learn in this book and keep your eye on the prize — losing up to 10 pounds!

The heart of the *Lose Up To 10 Pounds in 2 Weeks* program includes three basic steps:

1. Using a formula to determine the calories your body burns at rest, or your BMR

2. Tracking everything you eat and all the physical activity you do daily for 2 weeks

3. Creating a substantial daily calorie deficit — meaning that you are expending more calories than you take in through a combination of eating less and burning calories with exercise. The larger the calorie deficit you create each day, the more weight you will lose.

At the end of each day, you will add up the calories you ate and drank. Then you'll take the resulting number and subtract the calories burned from physical activity to calculate your Net Calories. Next, subtract your BMR (the calories your body burns at rest) to find your daily total calorie deficit. You can find a detailed example of this formula in the section called "Journal Pages."

In addition, with this program you will mentally create a calorie "budget" for each meal and snack, which means anticipating how many calories you need to save and preparing for each meal with a set amount to spend in mind. For example, you might budget 400 calories for lunch. You can have any meal and drink you want, as long as you stay within your budget. And, if it's possible to save a few calories by eating less than the budgeted amount, you can save up for the next meal or do slightly less exercise to lose even more weight!

If it sounds like a big change and hard work, that's because it is. No one is going to pretend it will be easy. You will have to make major changes, like cutting out empty carbs and calories, eating more fruits and vegetables and whole grains, and building fitness into your life every day. But the results will be worth it. Fitting into that favorite dress again, seeing the look on an old boyfriend's face, lounging on the beach in a swimsuit without feeling anxious — you will be highly rewarded for your hard work c ver the next 2 weeks and beyond.

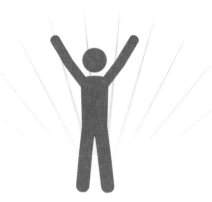

By purchasing this book, you have taken the first step in your weight-loss journey to looking and feeling amazing. In just 2 weeks, you could be 10 pounds lighter!

How to Use This Book

Congratulations! You've taken the first step toward losing real weight in a short amount of time by getting all the tools you need. Simply eating less or making a few foods swaps or spending some extra time at the gym isn't going to allow you to lose 10 pounds in only 2 weeks. People who think they can lose considerable weight without any help get frustrated and fail. This book offers you many valuable tools and features for cutting calories, getting in great shape, and successfully meeting your weight-loss goals, including:

Filling out your personal health and fitness profile

Before you begin the *Lose Up to 10 Pounds in 2 Weeks* program, you need to build Your Personal Profile. This section helps you assess your current physical state, habits, and preferences for diet and exercise. With this information, you will be able to determine where you started and how far you've come, as well as identify your goals and any potential obstacles.

In this section you will also determine the optimum amount of calories, fat and carbs that you will aim to eat every day.

Determining your BMR and creating a daily calorie deficit

An important part of the *Lose Up To 10 Pounds in 2 Weeks* program is calculating your basal metabolic rate, or BMR. Your BMR is the number of calories your body would burn naturally, even if you didn't move all day. Knowing this number is the first step to this program because it's how you build a calorie deficit.

Each day, you will total up the amount of calories you have eaten and subtract the calories you have burned from physical activity to find your Net Calorie Total. In order to lose up to 10 pounds in 2 weeks, you need to create a substantial calorie deficit each day, through a combination of diet and exercise. For example, one day, you may be able to cut 500 calories out of your diet, and then also burn 500 calories through exercise to create a 1,000-calorie deficit. Once you create a 3,500-calorie deficit, you will have lost 1 pound.

Powerful diet secrets and tips, fast places to trim calories, motivational quotes, and more

Each chapter and section of this book is packed with the secrets of cutting calories, making lifestyle changes, and losing weight. You will learn to boost your metabolism, make healthier eating decisions, as well as one of the best weight-loss strategies around: developing a game plan for avoiding pitfalls and sticking to your daily calorie goals. Throughout this book you will practice conscious eating, curb your appetite, and stop sabotaging your weight-loss efforts. You will also learn to anticipate and recognize situations that cause you to binge or eat unhealthy foods and pinpoint the emotions and triggers that cause you to overeat.

You will recognize the changes you can make without starving or depriving yourself, because no diet and fitness plan is going to work if you're feeling lethargic and hungry all the time. Burning hundreds of calories more than you take in a day might sound difficult, that's why each chapter in this book is complete with Did You Know facts, motivational quotes, and quick and easy places to trim 100, 200, and 300 or more calories. You'll discover new ways to eat less and lose weight that you never even thought of!

Finally, the diet section ends with 100 at-a-glance principles for losing weight. Any time you need a quick reminder for how to eat smart, make healthy diet swaps, or maintain motivation, flip back to this section to read the diet secrets at-a-glance.

Ultimate fitness secrets for burning calories and body fat and staying motivated

Fitness is going to be the second key to losing up to 10 pounds in this short amount of time. You can't do it with diet alone! These chapters will give you all the tips, tricks and tools to maximize each and every workout and physical activity you do. You'll get insight into everything from fitness basics to little-known secrets of getting in shape quickly and without burning out.

In the Activities & Calories Burned chapter, you'll see that calories are burned in all sorts of ways, from sports to casual physical activity to normal household chores. This section that will be a great asset in finding the sports and activities that you can make a part of your daily routine to burn calories.

Powerful 14-day exercise program for maximum weight loss

The fitness section also includes a detailed exercise program that combines a strength training circuit with a cardio circuit six days out of the week to burn calories and body fat quickly. The plan is designed to be done anywhere, so you won't need any props or weights. You will switch off each day between an upper body and core strength training circuit and a lower body and core strength training circuit. Each day, you will also alternate between a plyometric cardio circuit and a kickboxing cardio circuit. The last day of the week is to rest, recuperate and relax.

Finally, the fitness section ends with at-a-glance secrets for exercise and living an active, healthy life. The goal is to make physical activity a part of your everyday life — something you even look forward to. Refer to the secrets for getting fit in this section when you need a reminder of how to incorporate exercise and fitness into your day.

Reusable grocery list of healthy foods

Stop wandering the aisles of the supermarket, wondering what to buy to keep you and your family eating right. The *Lose Up To 10 Pounds in 2 Weeks* grocery list in the front of the book tears out to bring to the store and is laminated so it can be used again and again with a dry-erase marker.

This list takes the guesswork out of shopping by providing you with a comprehensive list of healthy, diet-smart products and food items by category — everything from fresh and canned produce to beverages to sweet treats! You can even write in your own supermarket favorites as you discover them. Even with this helpful list, don't forget to read the nutritional labels on all products.

Turn your high-calorie favorites into healthy meals with ingredient swaps

You'll never have to give up your favorite foods, such as fish and chips, tacos and pizza — simply use the healthy ingredient substitutions in the Make the Right Meal chapter. Take a look at the high calorie count of the original recipe, opt for the *Lose Up To 10 Pounds in 2 Weeks* version instead, and you'll save hundreds of calories while still eating the delicious meals you love. Losing weight shouldn't mean deprivation or going cold turkey from your favorite foods; the key is eating smarter in smaller portions and building your own healthy versions of the snacks, sides and entrées you crave.

Learn to order the right meals when dining out to save hundreds of calories

Dieters consistently say that dining out is one of the toughest obstacles to losing weight. That's because most restaurant menus have a very limited number of healthy, low-calorie choices. And while fast-food and the drive-thru window are cheap and convenient, you won't be doing your waistline any favors. The Order the Right Meal at America's Most Popular Restaurants chapter provides an at-a-glance look at the best and worst menu items for each category for approximately 140 of the country's most popular restaurants and fast-food chains. You'll never be stuck wondering what to order to stay within your intake goals again!

Use your number one weight-loss tool!

People who keep a food and fitness journal are proven to lose *twice* as much weight as those who don't. As you read all the valuable, powerful weight-loss and fitness tips in this book, you will be keeping track of what you eat and drink in the journal in the back of the book. Each daily page lets you write down the food and beverages you have daily, as well as the physical activities you do to burn calories. You'll easily be able to see what you've eaten and, thus, plan ahead for each meal and workout.

Keeping a diet journal will most likely be a healthy reality check. Studies have shown that people tend to dramatically underestimate the number of calories in the foods they eat — by as much as 50 percent! The diet and fitness journal portion of this book allows you to break down your caloric intake by meal and item to get real about exactly how many calories you're consuming. Once you recognize the high-calorie foods in your diet, you can replace some things with lower calorie options or cut back on portion sizes. Additionally, having your food intake right in front of you keeps you accountable — because who wants to look back and see the hundreds of calories from a pizza-and-cheese-bread binge written in their journal? You'll think twice before indulging in a huge or highly caloric meal. The journal will also help keep you motivated to exercise daily and provide a place to record your weight as the numbers on the scale begin to drop.

What happens after the 2 weeks?

Fast-forward 2 weeks: You've lost up to 10 pounds by following the diet and exercise program in this book! But now what? You can't just fall back into your old habits. You've worked too hard to put the weight right back on. This chapter gives you the secrets to making long-lasting changes that make exercising and eating smart a lifestyle and not just a short-term weight-loss experience. And every time you need a reminder of the best, most proven ways to be healthy, have energy, and make smart food choices, you should refer back to this book. Keep using a diet and fitness journal, your healthy eating grocery list, the restaurant guide, and the nutrition facts in this book to keep dropping unwanted pounds.

Nutritional information for more than 1,000 foods right at your fingertips!

Do you know how many calories are in your banana, egg salad, or glass of wine? Probably not, but the Nutrition Facts section in the back of this book will allow you to look up the calories, fat, carbs, protein and fiber for more than 1,000 common food items. Transfer these amounts into your diet journal to accurately keep track of your daily intake.

Your Personal Profile

Begin your program by gathering some information to assess your current physical state, habits, and preferences.

Fill in the information on the following pages. Visit your primary care physician and have your cholesterol, triglycerides, and blood pressure measured. These levels will also factor into the choices you make when creating your diet and fitness plan. You should also take your current measurements and place a "Before" photo in this section. It will be motivating to look back and see a visual of where you began and how far you have come.

Next, assess your diet and fitness history. You will also answer some questions about your past attempts to lose weight and what obstacles you encountered. Finally, outline your goals. Determine what you hope to accomplish with this program, which types of physical activities you most enjoy, and your intake goals, including the specific amounts of calories, fats, and carbs your diet should include daily.

Good luck meeting all your goals!

Your Health Profile

Complete the following personal health profile. You can request necessary information from your primary health care provider.

Name:_____   Triglycerides:_____

Age:_____   HDL Cholesterol:_____

Height:_____   LDL Cholesterol:_____

Total cholesterol:_____   Blood Pressure:_____

Current Physical Activity: (sedentary, moderately active, very active)

_____

_____

_____

_____

Current Diet & Eating Habits: (fast food, snack often, late-night eating, etc.)

_____

_____

_____

_____

Other Current Habits: (smoking, drinking, lack of sleep, etc.)

_____

_____

_____

_____

DATE:_____ WEIGHT:_____ BODY FAT %:_____

MEASUREMENTS:

[____] chest   [____] biceps   [____] waist   [____] hips   [____] thighs

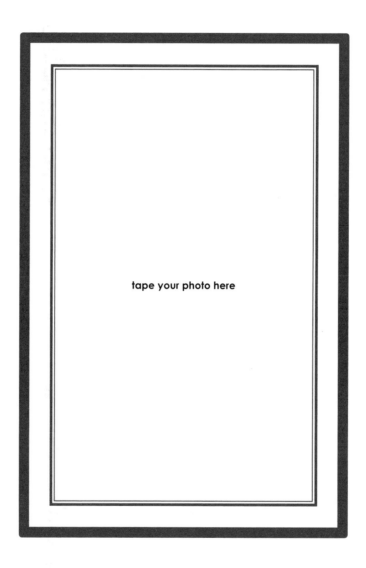

tape your photo here

PHOTO COMMENTS: _____

Dietary Habits Questionnaire

The following questions will assist you in developing your weight-loss program.

Which best describes your daily eating habits?
- ❏ Three average meals
- ❏ Graze frequently
- ❏ One large meal, little else

What types of food do you crave the most?
- ❏ Meat/fish
- ❏ Fruit/vegetables
- ❏ Bread/cereals/rice
- ❏ Sweets

Do you typically eat out or prepare food for yourself?
- ❏ I usually cook my food
- ❏ I eat out or have premade meals

What is your weight-loss goal?
- ❏ Lose 10 or more pounds
- ❏ Maintain weight
- ❏ Lose a little weight
- ❏ Improve health

Which habits do you have?
- ❏ Skipping meals
- ❏ Drinking full-sugar soda
- ❏ Carb addiction
- ❏ Overeating while dining out

Describe your body type:
- ❏ Overweight
- ❏ Average
- ❏ Muscular

For what particular event (if any) do you want to lose weight?

_____

_____

_____

_____

_____

_____

_____

What is your number one reason for wanting to lose weight?

_____

_____

_____

_____

_____

_____

_____

Your Diet & Intake Goals

A huge part of your weight-loss journey will be managing your diet and intake. Record your goals here and use them as a barometer for what you eat every day.

YOUR DIET GOALS

_____

_____

_____

_____

_____

_____

_____

_____

YOUR INTAKE GOALS

Based on the number of calories your diet allows, list the daily targets that you would like to meet. (Your primary care physician can also help you determine the appropriate amounts.)

DAILY CALORIES: FAT gms: CARBS gms: OTHER: _____

NOTES: _____

_____

_____

_____

_____

_____

Your Fitness History

It is important to look back at your past experiences with getting in shape and losing weight to determine the diet and workout plan that will have the greatest chance for success.

Is there any reason why you should not engage in physical activity?

_____

At what age were you in your best physical shape?

_____

Have you ever participated in a workout program? When?

_____

How long did you stay with the program?

_____

What did the program include?

_____

What led you to or inspired you to get into shape now?

_____

What obstacles have kept you from meeting your fitness goals?

_____

What will ensure these obstacles do not inhibit you this time?

_____

Rate your current fitness level on a scale of 1-10 (1=Worst 10=Best).

_____

Workout Plan Questionnaire

A successful fitness plan is one that includes activities you enjoy. Be honest in answering the following questions and you will be able to develop a plan you can maintain.

Which types of physical activity do you enjoy participating in?

- ☐ Aerobics
- ☐ Active gardening
- ☐ Backpacking
- ☐ Baseball/softball
- ☐ Bicycling/spinning
- ☐ Climbing
- ☐ Cross country skiing
- ☐ Dancing
- ☐ Downhill skiing
- ☐ Football
- ☐ Golfing
- ☐ Hiking
- ☐ Hockey
- ☐ Jogging/running
- ☐ Jump roping

- ☐ Martial arts
- ☐ Pilates
- ☐ Racquetball/handball
- ☐ Roller blading
- ☐ Rowing
- ☐ Soccer
- ☐ Skating
- ☐ Stair/bench stepping
- ☐ Stretching
- ☐ Swimming
- ☐ Tennis
- ☐ Volleyball
- ☐ Walking
- ☐ Weight training
- ☐ Yoga

How many times a week do you want to work out?

☐ 1-2 days   ☐ 2-3 days   ☐ 3-4 days   ☐ 5+ days

How long will each session be, on average?

- ☐ 10-20 minutes
- ☐ 20-30 minutes
- ☐ 30-45 minutes

- ☐ 45-60 minutes
- ☐ 60-90 minutes
- ☐ 90+ minutes

Your Fitness Goals

By first identifying your goals, you can create a specific workout routine to help you achieve them. Your goals should be specific, quantifiable, realistic and time-based. Fill out the following questions honestly and with a critical eye. You'll be able to use the resulting information to get inspired and ward off possible pitfalls.

What do you want to accomplish with your workout program? (Check the boxes next to the goals that are most important to you.)

☐ Improve cardiovascular fitness and endurance

☐ Improve diet and or eating habits

☐ Improve flexibility

☐ Improve health

☐ Improve strength

☐ Improve muscle tone and shape

☐ Increase energy

☐ Lose weight

☐ Prevent injury and/or rehabilitate injury

☐ Train for a sports-specific event

☐ Reduce cholesterol

☐ Reduce blood pressure

☐ Reduce risk of disease

☐ Reduce stress

☐ Gain weight

☐ Other: _____

☐ Other: _____

What types of physical activity do you like and dislike?

_____

_____

_____

_____

Do you prefer to exercise alone, with a partner, or in a group?

_____

_____

_____

_____

Calculating Your BMR

Knowing your basal metabolic rate, or BMR, is crucial to this program. Your BMR is the number of calories your body burns naturally, at rest. Your BMR is based on your age, height and current weight and decreases with age, meaning that it becomes harder to lose weight and keep it off as you get older. However, with a healthy diet and fitness plan, you can increase your BMR and lose weight more easily.

Use these formulas to calculate your BMR, then use this number in your daily diet and fitness journal pages.

Female BMR = 655 + (4.3 x weight in pounds) + (4.7 x height in inches) - (4.7 x age in years)

Male BMR = 66 + (6.3 x weight in pounds) + (12.9 x height in inches) - (6.8 x age in years)

Your BMR:

❝ The great thing in the world is not so much where we stand, as in what direction we are moving. **❞**

~ Oliver Wendell Holmes

Chapter 1

Changing the Way You Live

Losing weight takes a tremendous effort. If it were an easy thing to do, everyone would be at their perfect weight. When you talk about a body and lifestyle makeover, you can feel yourself getting excited, but when it comes time to actually implement the changes, your to-do list feels so long that you get overwhelmed and give up. Or, in the past you might have made it a few weeks into a weight-loss plan, failed to see results and quit. It's natural for the body to resist change. Your body tries to protect itself by slowing its basal metabolism, the rate at which you burn calories while at rest, making weight loss difficult. However, this program will have you looking and feeling better immediately, starting with the simple lifestyle changes in the chapter. Read through them and commit yourself to implementing them. They are what your body and mind need to jumpstart your weight loss, give you more energy, and get you motivated to complete the 2-week program.

Mahatma Gandhi once said, "Be the change you want to see in the world." Being healthier and living better are goals everyone should strive for. You will likely find that after living the *Lose Up To 10 Pounds in 2 Weeks* program, you won't want to stop! You'll feel better and slimmer than ever before, and you won't want to go back to old habits that packed on the extra pounds. However, even if you don't continue beyond this 2-week program, know that all the changes you'll find in this book are sustainable for a lifetime. This book gives you the tools to lose 10 pounds in 2 weeks, and more, including powerful, proven diet and exercise secrets and tips, motivational quotes, a healthy eating shopping list, restaurant guide, healthy meal guide, nutrition facts for common foods, and, the ultimate weight-loss tool, a daily diet and fitness journal. With all this at your fingertips, it's just up to you to put everything into practice.

Losing up to 10 pounds in 2 weeks starts by modifying your everyday habits. Today, you get a clean slate to erase the past and create a new, healthier, thinner way of living.

Keep your eye on the prize

Staying motivated is all about determining the top reasons you want and need to lose weight and reminding yourself on the days you're tempted to eat a high-calorie dessert or skip the gym. Are you losing weight to look and feel great at a special event that is 2 weeks away, such as a high school reunion, wedding, vacation or birthday? Or did your doctor advise you that losing 10 pounds will help reduce your risk of disease, lower your blood pressure, or help you get pregnant? Are you looking forward to the increased amount of energy you'll have after losing a few pounds? Or are you simply tired of feeling powerless to food? Make a short list of the top 3 reasons you are losing 10 pounds. Hang this list where you can see it every day to remind you, along with a motivational image — a gorgeous beach, a dress you'd like to buy in a smaller size, the hike you plan to take when you have more energy.

This book gives you the tools to lose up to 10 pounds in 2 weeks, and more, including powerful, proven diet and exercise secrets and tips, motivational quotes, a healthy eating shopping list, restaurant guide, healthy meal guide, nutrition facts for common foods, and, the ultimate weight-loss tool, a daily diet and fitness journal.

Create great new habits

Changing the way you live starts with building new, healthy habits that support your weight loss. Let's say you have the bad habit of eating empty-calorie candy and chocolate — replace it with a healthy habit. Instead of snacking on a candy bar when you are in the mood for something sweet, try having a 60-calorie pudding cup or a bowl of fresh strawberries with low-fat Cool Whip. Get in the habit of keeping those items in your kitchen instead of sugary snacks and you'll have made one awesome, positive change to your lifestyle! Focus on including the good behavior into your routine every day for a week until it becomes second nature.

Eat from all 6 of the main food groups

There are six main food groups: grains, fruits, vegetables, dairy, meat and beans, and oils and sweets. Odds are, you've been overdoing it in some and avoiding others all together. For instance, less than 3.5 percent of American men and women eat the FDA-recommended amount of fruits and vegetables. Unfortunately, when food groups are short-changed, you do not receive the balance of protein, carbohydrates, and plant-based nutrients that your body needs. To kickstart a sluggish metabolism, maintain your energy and inspire the body to burn fat cells, you must eat a balanced diet. The better you eat, the better your body works and the faster you'll lose weight. And you'll find that it only takes a few short days for your body to stop craving fatty and sugary processed foods. Some foods that pack mega-nutrients include low-fat yogurt, spinach, salmon, berries, avocados, whole grains, bell peppers, and olive oil.

Ransack your kitchen and pantry

Step 1: Get a big trash bag. Step 2: Open your cabinets, pantry, fridge and yes, even the hidden spots where you stash treats. Step 3: Throw every high-calorie, high-fat, sugary, salty, processed piece of food into your trash bag. Step 4: Take one last look in the bag before you toss the bag into a dumpster. Say goodbye to unhealthy, bloating, weight-gain-causing snacks and treats! Step 5: Feel inspired by your clean (perhaps nearly empty) cupboards and shelves. You now have a clean slate to start filling your kitchen with healthy foods. Likewise, cravings are very visual, so if you open your cupboards and don't see fatty foods, you won't constantly think about them.

Break the addiction to high-calorie food!

Did you realize that constantly treating yourself to high-calorie foods can lead to an actual addiction to these foods? Eating a high-calorie meal triggers the release of dopamine and other feel-good chemicals in the brain.

However, a ground-breaking report from the 2009 meeting for the Society for Neuroscience showed that rats that were fed a high-calorie diet of items like bacon, sausage and cheesecake actually had diminished response in the pleasure centers of their brains over time. As the animals' brain reward circuits became less responsive, they continued to overeat and become more and more obese. Their brains actually began to mimic those of rats addicted to drugs as they became addicted to high-calorie foods! Break this cycle by eliminating these high-fat, high-calorie foods from your grocery list. If they're not in the house or in your desk, you won't be tempted. Don't even look at the dessert list at a restaurant. Simply imagining yourself eating a delicious crème brulee can trigger an intense craving.

Get some shuteye

Research has proven that adults who get 7 to 9 hours of sleep a night eat less during the day and are much less likely to be overweight. For one, when you're sleep-deprived the body produces more of the hormone that causes feelings of hunger. Being exhausted also means less willpower to resist the temptation of fatty and sugary foods.

> One study showed that lack of sleep can lead to eating an extra 900 calories a day.

One study showed that lack of sleep can lead to eating an extra 900 calories a day. Wow! Consider that cutting those 900 calories a day for a year would mean a weight loss of more than 90 pounds! To lose up to 10 pounds in 2 weeks, you need to give your body the rest it needs. Try going to bed earlier and establishing a routine at night that is calming and gets you ready for deep sleep. For instance, things like being online or watching TV can disrupt your ability to fall asleep and stay asleep, so try reading for 30 minutes or taking a relaxing bath.

Back away from the TV

The National Weight Control Registry (NWCR) is an organization that studies the behavioral and psychological factors that contribute to weight loss and the maintenance of long-term weight loss. The NWCR tracks more than 5,000 individuals over the age of 18 who have maintained at least a 30-pound weight loss for one year or longer (although the average registry member has lost an average of 66 pounds and kept it off for 5.5 years), and found that there are a few common threads among members. About 80 percent of members report eating breakfast daily and, naturally, almost all members report continuing to maintain a low-calorie, low-fat diet and doing high levels of activity but, additionally, 62 percent say they watch less than 10 hours of TV per week. By contrast, the average American watched 38 hours a week, almost 4 times that much. That's nearly as many hours as a full-time job!

Obviously, if you're spending numerous hours a day in front of the TV, you're not exercising. In addition, vegging out leads to overeating of unhealthy foods, out of boredom or for comfort. Who ever curled up on the couch with a salad? As National Weight Control Registry members prove, getting off the couch and away from the TV aids in real weight loss. You'll eat less, and the hours you were spending watching a *Friends* marathon can now be spent hitting the gym, going for a walk with a friend, or otherwise being active outdoors.

Drink little to no alcohol

Alcohol makes losing 10 pounds in 2 weeks much tougher. For one, when you drink alcohol, that is what your body processes first, before fat, protein or carbs. Thus, alcohol slows down the fat-burning process. Also, a serving of alcohol contains at least 120 calories, and that number can skyrocket if you use sugary mixers. If you take in 120 calories from alcohol, you'll have to find another place to cut it, either with extra exercise or eating less at another meal. That can be very difficult since you're already going to be on a calorie-restricted diet.

Since the goal of this diet plan is to find fast and easy places to cut hundreds of calories, drinking alcohol is counterproductive. Plus, it's never smart or healthy to replace nutritious food with alcohol, which offers no nutrients.

Studies have shown as much as a 20 percent increase in calories consumed at a meal when alcohol was served beforehand.

Also, liquids don't satisfy you or fill you up. In fact, alcohol does quite the opposite. Research has shown that alcohol not only decreases willpower, it may stimulate the appetite — specifically cravings for fatty and salty foods. Studies have shown as much as a 20 percent increase in calories consumed at a meal when alcohol was served beforehand. So, while it's tough to say no alcohol at all for 2 weeks, the argument against it is very strong. Most dieticians believe there is no place for alcohol in a reduced-calorie diet.

"If you do not change direction, you may end up where you are heading."

~ Lao Tzu

Chapter 2

Maximizing Your Metabolism

We often hear about metabolism and its importance in helping us lose weight. But what exactly is metabolism, and how can you make yours work harder for you?

Metabolism is a series of chemical reactions that convert the food we eat into energy. This energy powers everything we do, from thinking to moving, healing, growing, and even aging. When you eat, you take in energy in the form of sugars (carbohydrates), proteins, and fats. But the body's cells cannot use energy in this form. So the body must break down these substances so the energy can be distributed to and used by the body's cells. Molecules in the digestive system called enzymes break down each substance differently: proteins are broken down into amino acids, fats are broken down into fatty acids, and carbohydrates are broken down into simple sugars, such as glucose. The process of breaking these substances down and using them for energy is metabolism.

Metabolism is a complicated chemical sequence, so it is easier to think of it in its most basic sense — metabolism is process that influences how easily you can gain and lose weight, or how easily you store or burn calories. The number of calories you are able to burn in a day depends on how high or low your metabolism is. Earlier in this book, you calculated your basal metabolic rate, or BMR. This is the rate at which your body burns calories while at rest. Everyone has a different BMR, which is largely inherited. You have probably heard friends lament, "Oh, I have the slowest metabolism in the world," or, "Have you seen how much so-and-so eats? She must have a super-fast metabolism." However, genetics don't determine everything when it comes to how quickly or slowly your body burns calories. You can actually change your BMR by doing certain activities and eating certain foods. For example, regular exercise can increase your body's BMR. Muscle burns 3 times as many calories as fat — about 6 calories per pound for muscle and only 2 calories per pound for fat. Therefore, every extra pound of muscle you put on burns 30 to 50 extra calories per day. Finally, your eating habits — the times at which you eat and your intake of protein or other metabolism-friendly foods — can also increase your BMR.

> If you're trying to subsist on carrots, lettuce and chicken soup, you'll be too exhausted to do much of anything but sit on the couch.

Don't settle for a slow metabolism or use it as an excuse for why you can't lose weight. This chapter gives you all the tips and tricks for super-charging your metabolism, starting from the moment you wake up in the morning.

Eat breakfast

It's called "the most important meal of the day" for a reason, and eating breakfast is essential for weight loss. Your body is deprived of food during the night — you are literally taking a "break" to "fast." Consider that if you ate dinner the night before at 7 p.m., and you go all the way to lunch without eating, you'll have fasted for 17 hours or more! Your blood sugar will be extremely low, plus, when your body doesn't receive sufficient nutrients post-fast, it will function less efficiently. Eating a balanced breakfast jumpstarts your metabolism, helps you eat a normal portion at lunch, and provides blood-sugar stability that means more energy, brainpower and focus for your day. And no, a cup of coffee isn't breakfast. Whole grains, oats, peanut butter, fruit, low-fat yogurt, and eggs are all good ways to start your day. They get your metabolism kicking and prevent overeating throughout the day.

Never skip meals

Dieters make the mistake of believing that skipping meals will help them cut calories and lose weight. But when you skip a meal your system goes into starvation mode. Your metabolism slows down to conserve energy and your body prepares to store fat during your next meal. Additionally, going too many hours between meals means you'll be so hungry the next time you eat that you'll eat far too much. Don't confuse your body by skipping meals; instead, eat small portions throughout the day. Try having three small meals and two or three healthy snacks throughout your day. This keeps your metabolism revved and working continuously and avoids blood sugar surges and crashes.

Eat small meals throughout the day

Increase your total calorie-burning capacity by having small, portion-controlled meals throughout the day. The act of eating helps increase your metabolism. The process of absorbing food requires energy. You burn calories with every meal as your body digests food. Keep your metabolism doing its job by spreading out large meals into smaller ones consumed throughout the day. You will end up burning more calories while still eating the same amount of food.

Eat enough!

Ensure that you are eating enough to keep your metabolism active. Many people mistakenly believe that if they reduce their caloric intake to a very low amount, such as 1,000 calories a day, they'll be able to lose weight more quickly. However, your body and organs, such as the heart, kidneys and liver, need a certain amount of calories simply to function, much less to get you through a day at work, playing with your kids, and exercising. If you're trying to subsist on carrots, lettuce and chicken soup, you'll be too exhausted to do much of anything but sit on the couch, and you'll never lose real weight. Find a healthy balance that lets you lose weight but provides enough energy as well.

Did You Know?

While you may have inherited your metabolism from Mom and Dad, it doesn't mean you can't do some things to give a slower metabolism a big boost. Increasing your muscle mass; eating high-protein, low-fat, low-calorie meals and snacks throughout the day; never skipping meals; and being physically active all speed it up naturally!

Never go too long without eating

Waiting too long between meals can slow down the rate at which your body burns fat, as well as cause blood sugar dips that lead to overeating feeling sluggish. Instead, try eating every 3 or 4 hours and choose nutritious foods — light cheese and whole grain crackers, small salads, hummus and vegetables, peanut butter on whole wheat toast, baked fish and chicken — and you won't overindulge at any one meal. Keep healthy snacks handy for those days when you're away from your office or house and won't have time to fix something. You never want to go more than 4 hours without putting energizing food in your system.

Drink coffee and green tea

Coffee can be a helpful diet tool as it suppresses hunger and kick-starts the metabolism. Research shows that green tea can actually help you burn fat and increase your metabolism. Green tea contains very special compounds called catechin polyphenols. These antioxidants help you drop pounds by increasing fat oxidation and thermogenesis, the process where your body temperature increases as a result of burning fat. Green tea can also prevent the storage of excess sugar and fat in the body. Another antioxidant, epigallocatechin gallate (EGCG) has been proven effective at regulating glucose levels which may help reduce your appetite. Drinking 5 cups of green tea may burn 70 to 80 extra calories a day.

> Drinking 5 cups of green tea may burn 70 to 80 extra calories a day.

Stay hydrated!

Maintaining hydration is crucial for weight loss. Water keeps your metabolism working hard, maintains digestion, improves muscle tone, and makes your stomach feel full. Try having a tall glass of water shortly before every meal. How much should you drink? You need to drink at least eight 8-ounce glasses a day. That's the minimum! Men should really strive for 120 ounces of water and women should try and get 90 ounces. If you think about it, it's really not a lot. Buy a regular 750-ml aluminum water bottle (available at any store from Target to Starbucks to your local gym) and fill it up three times and you've already had more than eight glasses. No matter what your ideal water consumption is, remember to increase water intake in conditions such as high heat, high altitude, low humidity, or high activity level. Water is necessary in order for metabolism to take place, so being properly hydrated helps your body turn food into the energy you need for work, family and exercise.

Eat spicy foods

Some research suggests that spicy foods, primarily red pepper, cayenne, and chili pepper, may help raise your metabolism. These foods may increase your calorie burning capacity for up to 2 to 3 hours after eating. The heat generated from capsaicin can increase your body temperature and temporarily raise your metabolic rate by around 8 percent. While studies need to prove whether or not this rate has a profound effect on weight loss, eating spicy foods may also help you lose weight by increasing feelings of satisfaction. The additional water needed to quench the heat from foods may also aid in feeling full when eating a spicy meal.

Men should strive for 120 ounces of water and women should try and get 90 ounces. Increase your intake in high heat, high altitude, low humidity, or high activity level.

Add lean protein to your diet

Proteins are building blocks for your body. Unlike fat and carbohydrates, which are primarily sources of energy, proteins play an important role in the function and repair of body tissues. Proteins help build muscles and can increase your metabolic rate. It takes more energy for your body to break down protein than it does carbohydrates or fat because of the increased "thermic" effect of digesting protein. In all, the energy it takes just to digest and absorb protein accounts for approximately 25 percent of the total calories protein contains. Ground turkey, skinless white meat poultry, as well as egg whites, fish, and legumes, are great sources of lean protein.

Eat "negative calorie" foods

Nutrient-rich, fiber-dense foods burn more calories than they contain. Even though fruits and vegetables have calories, they are referred to as "negative calorie" foods. Negative calorie foods usually contain high amounts of nutrients and fiber, and the high fiber content requires more energy to digest than the amount of calories in the food itself. Some negative calorie foods you can eat are asparagus, berries, broccoli, cucumbers, lettuce, grapefruit, oranges, melons, peaches, and plums.

The energy it takes to just digest and absorb protein accounts for approximately 25 percent of the total calories protein contains.

❝ When you come to the end of your rope,
tie a knot and hang on. **❞**

~ Franklin D. Roosevelt

Chapter 3

Secrets for Planning Ahead

Your life is packed with commitments that take time and energy, and this also makes it difficult to lose weight. If you are heading to an appointment around a mealtime, you will probably grab something prepackaged or from the drive-thru, rather than making something fresh and healthy. After a long workday, having pizza and breadsticks delivered to your house sounds much more appealing than cooking a nutritious meal. Or, you might skip out on going to the gym when a friend calls and wants to meet for dinner and drinks. Indeed, work, school, errands, family, friends, and other daily tasks constantly threaten to derail us from working out and eating right. Unless you specifically plan to build healthy habits into your daily life, the best-laid intentions will fall by the wayside. As long ago as 400 B.C., Chinese philosopher Confucius wrote, "When it is obvious that the goals cannot be reached, don't adjust the goals, adjust the action steps." The way you have been living, sacrificing your weight and health in favor of other commitments, is not working. It is critical for the success of this diet program that you don't leave healthy eating to chance. Develop a game plan for how to avoid pitfalls and stick to your healthy habits.

Planning ahead, in spite of a busy or stressful schedule, can make all the difference between losing 10 pounds in 2 weeks and not losing any weight. Determine ahead of time what you will eat at each meal. Build a repertoire of healthy recipes and stock basic ingredients so you'll never be left wondering what to eat. Be prepared with healthy snacks. Make a mental list of the fast-food items you can eat without blowing your calorie count. Treat plans to exercise as appointments that cannot be rescheduled.

Burning or saving an extra 500, 1,000 or 2,000 calories a day will be a challenge already, so you need to plan properly to make the best food and fitness choices you can. Use the following principles to create a successful game plan for cooking, dining out, creating a calorie budget, and more.

Make a list of all the healthy foods you enjoy

Facing the reality that you'll need to create a substantial calorie deficit each day for the next 2 weeks can be overwhelming and daunting. You may feel like there is nothing you can eat when you are trying to lose weight. Make grocery shopping and planning meals easier by writing a complete list of the healthy foods you enjoy. Once you write down all the foods you love that you can still include in your reduced-calorie diet, your options will seem a lot broader and more appealing. Consider the recommended low-fat and low-calorie dairy products, cereal, meat and seafood, soup and canned goods, frozen meals, salad dressings, prepackaged snacks, beverages, treats, and more from the tear-out shopping list in the beginning of this book, and write down your own favorites.

Plan your meals for the entire week

Don't wait until Monday evening when your stomach is growling to try and decide what to cook for dinner. Use your weekend to plan your menu for the following week. If [...] u are already in the mindset t[...] e less likely to use the weeke[...] t your schedule for the week [...] y meals, based on the amou[...] o the store to purchase all t[...] e yourself a quick, healthy lu[...] k salads with grilled chicken [...] soup and half a turkey sa[...] y veggies. Preparing for the [...] y and making your own me[...] hundreds of calories per me[...]

Handwritten note:

- Fish   - sandwiches
chicken   rice/protein/veggies
- Turkey   - Turkey sandwiches
- Brocoli
- cauliflower
- rau moun
- cereal - cherrios

Make a menu every week
- Sunday ——>
~~appetizers~~
split the entree

Know your "calorie budget" for each meal

will fall by the wayside.

Practice planning ahead by budgeting your calories at each meal. By writing everything you eat or drink in your journal in the back of this book, you will know how many calories you have saved and how many you have to spend on each meal to reach your intake goals. Consider any starters (soup or salad, perhaps), your main course, sides and beverages. For example, have water: zero calories. Cross "beverages" off your list. Have a small side salad to start. Calories: 150. Have a 250-calorie turkey sandwich, hold the mayo, and you're at 400 calories. Now let's say you had budgeted 500 calories for this meal. You could spend that last 100 calories on a cookie, which provides a few moments of enjoyment, or you could save those last 100 calories. If you make this same choice every day at every meal and you will see the difference on the scale and in the mirror at the end of the week — guaranteed.

Have a game plan for dining out

A recent study showed that people consume 50 percent more calories, fat, and sodium when they eat out. But just because you're trying to lose up to 10 pounds in 2 weeks, doesn't mean you have to pass on dinner with friends — you just need to plan ahead so you don't overeat. According to Purdue University research, eating a pre-meal snack of a handful of peanuts about an hour before dinner will lead you to eat less total calories and fat during your main meal. Also, a broth-based soup or small side salad are good pre-meal choices. To eat less, anticipate what you're going to order, so your eyes don't get bigger than your stomach when you're sitting at the table with all your friends. Almost all restaurant menus are online now, and many also provide nutritional facts, so check ahead of time and decide what you're going to have. Consider ordering an appetizer, such as steamed mussels or a Caprese salad, as your meal. Restaurants are notorious for doubling and even tripling portion sizes, so truly, an appetizer or half-portion is probably all the food you need anyway.

Did You Know?

Research estimates that soft drinks make up between 5.5 and 7 percent of the calories in an American diet! If you haven't already, give up full-sugar soda immediately. However, simply drinking diet soda isn't enough of a weight-loss game plan. Be sure you're not ordering the fried chicken bucket just because you're enjoying a zero-calorie soda.

Start a recipe folder

When you're trying to decide what to cook, you need an array of healthy options right at your fingertips or you'll be tempted to call for take-out or pick up greasy fast-food. Start keeping a recipe folder. Go online and print out healthy recipes from sites like CookingLight.com or EatingWell.com. Or, buy magazines like *Real Simple* that offer fast, healthy recipes with complete calorie and fat information and fill your folder with tear-outs. Better still, contact friends and family who are in good shape and ask for their healthy, tried-and-true recipes. You could even start a healthy-recipe email chain that lots of people you know will benefit from.

Make a shopping list and stick to it

Focus on shopping for only the items you need to lose weight and stick to the list you made earlier in this chapter. Grocery stores stock the most tempting foods at eye level and in the center aisles. It's easy to get sidetracked if you let your eyes wander. It's also hard to resist a good bargain. Sale items can be difficult to pass up, so avoid the "endcaps" of store aisles, which offer low prices on processed items that have a high profit margin for the store, like donuts, sugary cereal, soda, chips and dip, and other unhealthy foods. You will be less susceptible to bright packaging, enticing deals, and other impulse items if you put on grocery shopping blinders and stick to your list.

> After a meal, you could spend your last 100 calories on a cookie, which provides a few moments of enjoyment, or you could save those last 100 calories. Save them and you will see the difference on the scale at the end of the week — guaranteed.

Don't grocery shop when you're hungry

Stores use merchandising tricks such as smell, product placement, overall store layout, and sale items to get you to buy more. These ploys encourage you to shop longer and spend more money. You may end up buying more food than you need, especially if you are hungry. Stop by the grocery store after a meal when you won't be as likely to stray from your shopping list. Or, drink a large glass of water. The feeling of fullness will make it easier to resist food. Another tip is to chew on a piece of peppermint gum while you shop. You will be less likely to try free samples.

Plan ahead for travel

If you travel often and will be spending a lot of time in airports and on planes in the next 2 weeks, you must have a strategy that enables you to still lose weight. In-flight snacks are typically chips and crackers, with 200 or more empty calories in each tiny package. Airport food is even worse — pre-made sandwiches, personal pizzas, burritos, and barbecue are common layover fare, so you're looking at up to 800 calories. Ward off extra calories by packing portable, healthy snacks in your carry-on when you are faced with layovers, long flights or possible delays. Raw, pre-cut veggies, an apple, dried fruits and nuts, and whole wheat crackers with natural peanut butter are easy-to-pack snacks. Or, make a sandwich (hold the mayo) that you wrap in tin foil and eat mid-flight. Other travelers will be jealous of your healthy, tasty meal!

Outsmart the minibar

A weary traveller can easily be tempted by the hotel minibar and its salty and sweet snacks that are just an arm's length away. Practice this celebrity trick and save hundreds of calories by calling your hotel ahead of time and asking that the minibar be locked up or emptied all together. It's too easy to give into temptation when you're on-the-go, so plan ahead for an out-of-town stay. Instead, bring healthy snacks with you or stop by a grocery store to stock up on smart options to keep in your room.

Keep meal replacement options in your car or desk

There are times when a fresh, home-cooked meal isn't an option, so have some meal replacement bars and shakes on hand. While they aren't a long-term meal substitute, they are certainly the better choice when you need nutrition in a hurry and your other choice is the drive-thru or vending machine. Stick to drinks and bars that provide a balanced 40/30/30 or 40/40/20 ratio of carbohydrates, fats, and proteins. Steer clear of bars with too many simple sugars, which add empty carbs and don't satiate you over an extended time period. Instead, look for a bar with more fiber, which will make you feel full longer. And stay away from anything that contains partially hydrogenated oils, which are a source of heart-clogging trans fats.

Cook and freeze meals for later

While fresh is always better than frozen, many busy people enjoy the fact that frozen meals save them time. If you like the efficiency and convenience of frozen diet meals, try taking one evening or weekend afternoon to make a large batch of fresh food that can be divided into servings, frozen, and reheated later. Soup, chili, and vegetarian lasagna are just a few great options that can be made in healthy ways. Store each portion in an airtight container, freeze, and enjoy for up to three months. Having a frozen pre-portioned meal on hand at all times means you won't be tempted to go for fast-food when you're short on time.

> Don't wait until Monday evening when your stomach is growling to try and decide what to cook for dinner. Use your weekend to plan your menu for the following week.

" Live to the point of tears. **"**

~ Albert Camus

Chapter 4

Curbing Your Appetite

Our need for food is first and foremost a biological need. Our body needs calories, fat, nutrients, vitamins, carbohydrates, water, and proteins to carry out complex biochemical reactions that allow us to grow, heal, and function. But of course, if eating were primarily about giving our bodies the energy they need to function, we would simply take a pill or gel that contained our daily nutritional values and call it a day. In reality, eating is a social activity often dictated by our desires for certain kinds of food.

This love of food, or what we call "appetite," however, causes us to eat when we are not hungry, to overeat because we like how a food tastes, to crave foods that are bad for us, and to substitute eating for other activities when we are bored or restless. Our love of eating causes us to forget the primary biological reasons we are supposed to eat. This, combined with technological advances in food preparation and preservation and a higher standard of living, provides us with a dizzying array of choices through which to satisfy our hungry stomachs.

Controlling your appetite is one of the most important parts of losing 10 pounds in 2 weeks. The best way to curb your appetite is to continually remind yourself that while eating is pleasurable, you should do so primarily because you have a physical need to eat. Food is fuel for your day, for exercise, for mental focus, and for your well-being.

Indulging in the bad foods you crave forms neuronal connections in the brain. When these pathways get constantly activated and reinforced you end up thinking about and craving those foods all the time.

The tips and secrets you learn in this chapter will help you determine what causes you to eat when you're not hungry, restrict your desire for food when your body does not really need it, stave off cravings for high-calorie foods, and eat less overall to lose weight.

Ask yourself, What type of hunger is this?

One key to losing weight is to identify your hunger and stop mindless snacking and eating. People may eat when they're not hungry or they overeat when they are extremely hungry and have low blood sugar. Sometimes people eat more in a social setting, surrounded by friends. Other times, they eat more sitting home alone, out of loneliness or boredom. One specific food may even trigger overeating. Since you cannot avoid food, you need to identify your hunger and find a way to address that need in the right way. Figure out if you are experiencing true physical hunger, low blood sugar hunger, cravings, comfort eating, or social hunger. Once you are honest with yourself about why you're eating, you can put down the chips and wait until you're experiencing true physical hunger to eat a full, healthy meal.

Know what foods trigger your appetite

Identify the foods that send your appetite out of control. These are foods that you find yourself compulsively overeating after one bite. Common trigger foods usually combine sugar and fat, or fat and salt. Binges are linked to the food itself; for example, if donuts are one of your trigger foods, a single bite can result in you eating 3 donuts, regardless of your hunger, situation, or emotional state. Until you are able to stop these impulses, you should avoid your trigger foods completely. Avoid even walking past the bakery section at the grocery store. Don't have a box of Girl Scout cookies at home if you know you won't stop with just one cookie. For now, skip the office happy hour if you know you'll be tempted to binge on salty bar food.

Recognize that seeing foods you crave makes you want them more

Your sense of sight is a key factor in controlling your appetite and losing weight. Research has shown that seeing and indulging in the bad foods you crave over and over forms neuronal connections in the brain. When these pathways get constantly activated and reinforced you end up thinking about and craving those foods all the time. When a person sees a food he or she likes, the brain becomes very active; on the flip side, brain waves show less activity when people look at foods they don't particularly like. Even a photo of a tasty dish can increase your appetite. Don't linger over menus with large images of high-calorie meals and don't even look over at the dessert tray. Don't let your gaze wander to other dinners when eating out. Simply recognizing that sight has a significant impact on your appetite will help you fight the temptation to eat when you are not hungry.

Steer clear of refined carbohydrates

Refined carbs are items made with sugars and white flour, such as white pasta, rice, bagels, donuts and muffins. Ever notice how your morning bagel actually makes you feel hungrier after you eat it? That's because the body processes refined carbs so quickly that your blood sugar surges and drops. When blood sugar levels drop, the body feels hungry. So, you've not only eaten a 450-calorie bagel with cream cheese, you're ready to eat again mid-morning. Stick to complex carbohydrates that are low in fat and provide healthy protein, such as oatmeal, whole grain rice, yams, beans and more. These foods slow the digestion process and the release of sugar into the bloodstream to keep levels stable and hunger at bay.

Did You Know?

You may have heard that red wine is high in healthy-giving antioxidants; however, don't use that as an excuse for drinking alcohol and derailing your weight loss. Red wine contains 120 calories a glass or more and alcohol is known to stoke the appetite. To benefit from antioxidants, try drinking green or black tea instead.

Alcohol may make you hungrier

A night of drinks and dinner may sound like a good time, but it's wreaking havoc on your weight loss. The first issue is that liquids don't satisfy you or fill you up. In fact, research has shown that alcohol not only decreases willpower, it whets the appetite and increases cravings for high-sodium, high-fat foods (consider traditional "bar food," which is things like onion rings, burgers, nachos, and hot wings). There can be as much as a 20 percent increase in calories consumed at a meal when alcohol was served beforehand. And with the calories from the alcohol added in, there is a 33 percent total increase in calories. Secondly, after a night of imbibing, the alcohol is what the body breaks down first, before other nutrients, slowing the fat-burning process. The bottom line is, don't drink and eat and you'll save hundreds of calories.

Slow down!

You eat quickly because of a hectic schedule, because you're on-the-go, or simply because you're a fast eater. However, studies show that people who eat quickly consistently overeat and tend to be more overweight than people who eat slowly. When you eat, your body releases hormones that indicate fullness and tell your brain that you are satisfied. It takes up to 20 minutes for this process to take be complete. During this time, it is very easy to stuff yourself with much more food than you really need if you're eating quickly. Use smaller utensils, take smaller bites, chew your food thoroughly, take a drink of water, and put your utensils down between bites. Try eating half of what's on your plate, wait 10 minutes, then have a few more bites if you're still hungry.

Go minty after meals

Studies have shown that mint flavor and smell may suppress appetite for a short period of time, so brush your teeth or chew a piece of mint gum after meals. The majority of what your brain perceives as taste is actually smell, so if you saturate your sense of smell with a strong odor, like mint, the smell of food will be less appealing and you're less likely to eat more than you need. In one study from Wheeling Jesuit University, 40 people sniffed peppermint every 2 hours for 5 days, then sniffed a placebo for the next 5 days. During the week they smelled the peppermint, they consumed 1,800 fewer calories. Also, if you are susceptible to nighttime snacking, brush your

A recent study showed that people consume 50 percent more calories, fat, and sodium when they eat out. Plan ahead so you don't overeat.

teeth early so you won't be tempted to snack after dinner. If you can, keep a travel-size toothbrush and toothpaste set with you in your car and at work.

Don't go cold turkey with cravings

Don't make your favorite foods off-limits, because you will immediately crave what you deny yourself. And succumbing to cravings leads to overeating. When you eat sweet, salty or high-calorie foods, your brain releases dopamine and other pleasure chemicals. When you deprive yourself of these foods, your body shifts into hedonism mode, demanding what makes it feel good. In addition, people have a tendency to want what they can't have, what is "forbidden." When you go cold turkey from your favorite foods, you dwell on thoughts of those more, until you give in to your craving and you binge. Instead, treat yourself but in a smart way. Eat pre-portioned amounts of the treats you crave, such as the 100-calorie packs of cookies, crackers and chips sold at all grocery stores. Everything from Reese's Peanut Butter Cups to Pringles now come in 100-calorie snack sizes. Allow yourself just one of these packages when the craving for something sweet or salty feels truly overwhelming.

Be the last person to start eating when dining out

People eat between 40 and 70 percent more food when eating in big groups. We tend to adopt the eating behaviors of the majority, no matter how unhealthy they may be. Be the last to start eating in groups in order to lose weight and keep calories down. Also, recognize that social interactions within groups of people tend to lengthen mealtimes. Longer mealtimes increase the likelihood that you will eat more. Don't feel the need to keep up with the table and match each bite of other people's food with your own.

Mix up your routine

Altering your routine can help you avoid the triggers and temptations that cause hunger and overeating. If you typically meet a friend for drinks and appetizers after work on Fridays, this may be a routine that has to change.

Interestingly enough, the sights and smells of these familiar places may be triggering your compulsion to eat and not the foods themselves. Meet your friend for coffee one morning instead and order a flavored coffee without milk for a zero-calorie drink. Or, if driving past your neighborhood taco shop every day makes your stomach grumble thinking about mega-calorie burritos, take a different route. You can easily save 500 or more calorie just by curbing that craving.

The majority of what your brain perceives as taste is actually smell, so if you saturate your sense of smell with a strong odor, like mint, the smell of food will be less appealing.

ɛɛ Always bear in mind that your own resolution to succeed is more important than any other. **ɟɟ**

~ Abraham Lincoln

Chapter 5

Controlling Your Portions

A few years ago, the North American Association for the Study of Obesity performed a fascinating study on portion control and soup. Some of the 54 participants were given a regular bowl containing a regular portion of soup and asked to eat as much of it as they liked. Other participants, however, were given a self-refilling bowl of soup. Soup was automatically piped into the bottom of the bowl as the participants were eating, making it impossible for them to ever reach the bottom. Participants were not told that extra soup was being added to their portion, and the soup was piped in so slowly it was impossible for them to tell that soup was being added as they were eating it.

Researchers found that participants who ate from the self-refilling bowl ate a whopping 73 percent more than participants who ate from a normal bowl. Perhaps more astonishing was the fact that those who ate from the self-refilling bowls did not report feeling any more full than those who ate from the regular bowls. Furthermore, the study found that a person's weight did not affect whether they were likely to keep eating from the self-refilling bowls. Participants eating from the self-refilling bowls included overweight, normal weight, and underweight participants. Across the board, everyone ate more, no matter what their weight or mood.

This study proved what most people have already come to realize: the size of your portion determines how much you will eat, regardless of how hungry you are.

Another interesting study of the factors that lead to over-consumption, published in the *Journal of Consumer Research* in 2008, found that a concept called "extremeness aversion" also contributes to bad portion control, overeating and obesity. Extremeness aversion is the tendency for individuals to avoid the smallest and largest sizes and order the middle size — no matter how large. According to Kathryn M. Sharpe, Richard Staelin and Joel Huber, authors of the study, this concept has gradually led retailers to offer larger and larger portions and consumers to choose larger and larger portions. You may have noticed that businesses like movie theaters and fast food restaurants have begun to inflate the sizes of highly caloric items like popcorn, fries and soft drinks. The study showed that if a fast-food restaurant originally offered 21-ounce, 16-ounce and 12-ounce options for soft drinks, most consumers would rule out the large and small sizes and choose the middle size, 16 ounces. However, when the restaurant eliminated the 12-ounce drink, consumers would choose the 21-ounce drink, because the 16-ounce drink they preferred earlier was now the smallest size, or the extreme, making it less desirable.
Additionally, studies have proven that people are terribly inaccurate when it comes to eyeballing correct portions. A study referenced in the *Journal*

of *Marketing Research* showed that consumers' perceptions of serving size are highly unreliable and can unknowingly vary as much as 20 percent. Another study showed that consumers vastly underestimate the caloric content of the foods they eat. In a recent study, researchers asked consumers to estimate the number of calories in different fast food meals. Most participants estimated 700 to 800 calories for these meals — about half of the actual amount.

Portion control is three-fold: being aware and anticipating situations in which you may be served large portions, eating smaller portions, and feel satiated by smaller portions. While this may not be easy at first, you will quickly learn that you can be perfectly happy with much less food than you have been eating. And it should be fairly easy to recognize the environments in which you are likely to overeat. For example, certain restaurants are well-known for serving outlandish portions — two and three times the amount you need to eat. Or you may be aware that visiting family means large meals with lots of food. Having a plan going into these situations can help you maintain proper portion control — and self-control.

Use these tips and secrets to keep your portions reasonable and your weight loss on track. Controlling your portion sizes is one of the very best ways to build a substantial calorie deficit each day.

Know the correct serving size for your favorite foods

Do you know what a single serving is for your favorite foods, such as pasta, chicken, rice, oatmeal, fruit and more? The reality of dieting is that you *can* eat most of the foods you love if you exercise portion control. First, that means educating yourself about what one serving of your favorite foods really is!

Keep in mind that certain factors affect food portions, such as the individual's age, gender and activity level, but according to the USDA, one serving equals:

- 1 slice of whole grain bread
- 1/2 cup of cooked rice or pasta
- 1/2 cup of mashed potatoes
- 3-4 small crackers
- 1 small pancake or waffle
- 2 medium-sized cookies
- 1/2 cup cooked vegetables
- 1/2 cup tomato sauce
- 1 cup lettuce
- 1 small baked potato
- 1 medium apple
- 1/2 grapefruit or mango
- 1/2 cup berries
- 1/3 cup dried fruit or nuts
- 2 tbsp peanut butter
- 1 cup yogurt or milk
- 1 1/2 ounces of cheese
- 1/2 cup dry beans
- 1/2 cup tofu
- 1 chicken breast
- 1 medium pork chop
- 1/4 pound hamburger patty
- 1 tsp butter or margarine

Learn to eyeball portion sizes

No need for annoying measuring cups or a food scale — a handful here and a scoop there ... that looked like a tablespoon, right? Wrong. Research has shown that people can't eyeball portions without some practice. You won't always have a measuring cup on-hand, and who knows what an ounce of something looks like? Create a system in which you associate the size of a familiar object, like a golf ball or your fist, to serving sizes of your favorite foods. You need to learn how to associate common objects with the serving size of foods. After some time, you will be able to recognize correct portions just by how they fill up a plate, bowl or pan. Here is a list to help you get started, or come up with your own serving-size associations if you like:

A way to put your frozen dinners to work for weight loss is to save the empty containers, then wash them out and use them as a model for proper portion sizes the next time you cook.

- Vegetables or fruit: the size of your fist or a baseball
- Pasta: one handful
- Meat, fish, or poultry: a deck of cards or the size of your palm
- Snacks (chips, pretzels, etc): a cupped handful
- Apple: a baseball
- Potato: a computer mouse
- Bagel: a hockey puck
- Pancake: a CD
- Ice cream: a tennis ball
- Steamed rice: a cupcake wrapper
- Cheese: size of your whole thumb
- Dried fruit or nuts: a golf ball or an egg
- Cereal: a fist
- Dinner roll: a bar of soap
- Peanut butter: a ping pong ball
- Butter or margarine: a postage stamp
- Salad dressing: a ping pong ball

Create a harmony between carbs, protein & veggies

A simple way to stick with moderate portions is to figure out the proportions of protein, carbohydrates, and vegetables for your meal. Divide your plate into halves. Start out by filling the first half of your plate with non-starchy vegetables, such as a salad, green beans, or grilled tomatoes. Fill a quarter of your plate with protein. Choose from fish, poultry, or lean cuts of beef. The other quarter should be a starchy vegetable or grain like sweet potatoes. Now you can ensure your meal is nutritionally balanced and that you'll feel full and satisfied.

Order single items rather than combo or meal deals

Create a system in which you associate the size of a familiar object, like a golf ball or your fist, to serving sizes of your favorite foods.

Fast food restaurants lure customers with combo meals that include a variety of items at a low price. Avoid these marketing ploys no matter how great the value. The amount of calories in a combo meal can contain more than a days worth of calories. For example, a quarter-pound cheeseburger, large fries, and a 21-ounce milkshake has over 1,800 calories. If you have to eat fast-food, you can still lose weight by creating your own combo. Places like McDonald's will let you make substitutions, such as apple slices for fries and grilled chicken for breaded and fried chicken. The kids' menu also often includes more reasonable portions.

Eat from smaller dishware and silverware

One trick that can help control portion size when you're eating at home is using smaller plates, bowls, glasses and silverware. Think about it: If you're using a large dinner plate, you're more inclined to fill it completely with spaghetti and meatballs — and eat the whole plate of food. But if you eat with smaller dishware, it gives the impression that there is more food or drink, so your brain will report that you're full and satisfied from a smaller portion. And using smaller spoons and forks means taking smaller bites, eating more slowly and enjoying your meal longer, giving your body time to feels satiated.

Stock your freezer with healthy frozen foods

If your freezer is full of healthy frozen entrees and frozen meats and vegetables, you won't be tempted to call for take-out or get fast-food when you're hungry. Check the reusable grocery list in this book to help you stock up on meals with up to 400 calories and less than 10 grams of fat, as well as items such as frozen peas, broccoli, spinach, berries, boneless and skinless chicken breasts, fish, shrimp, pork loin, ground turkey, and more. On the other hand, items to leave out of your freezer include ice cream, chocolate, alcohol and any other temptations.

Order a "bistro size" or "lunch portion" of salads and entrées. This portion size will leave you happy and full at the majority of restaurants.

Use frozen diet dinner trays for portion control

An awesome benefit of frozen diet meals is that they are nutritionally balanced, portion-controlled and provide an accurate idea of how much fat, carbs, sodium and calories you're eating. Another way to put your frozen dinners to work for weight loss is to save a few of the empty containers when you're done eating. Wash them out and use them as a model for proper portion sizes the next time you cook. Frozen diet meals can be an excellent teacher for understanding the right ratios of protein to vegetables to starch to sauce.

Don't put serving dishes out on the table

Part of losing weight and exercising portion control is feeling satiated from a smaller amount of food than you're used to. It's important to know that sense of satiation is very visual. If you set bowls or pans of food out on the table, you are simply encouraging yourself to take seconds. Serve yourself a reasonable portion size while you're in the kitchen, then put the rest of the food away for leftovers. This way you won't be tempted to take more of anything. Savor and appreciate each bite. After you eat, busy yourself with dishes and cleaning up your cooking space — this gives your brain a chance to register that your body is full, and you won't feel the need to grab another dinner roll or helping of potatoes.

Take the food out of its container

When you're eating out of a container, there is also a tendency to feel like you haven't eaten enough to satisfy you. If you take the food out of the packaging your brain will register just how much you're really eating.

People who include nuts in their diet often have lower risk of heart disease; however, enjoy them in moderation, because nuts are very calorie-dense.

A yogurt may not look like much in its packaging, but you'll discover its contents actually fill a bowl. And how many times have you gotten to the bottom of a 100-calorie snack pack and commented, "There were only four cookies in there!" If you pour them out ahead of time, your brain has a chance to register that you are, in fact, eating a full handful of small cookies, which is a healthy portion for losing weight.

Order the smallest size meal when dining out

We all know that portion control is much easier when we're eating at home. At home we can regulate how much we put on a plate, whereas at a restaurant, portions are often two and even three times the size of what we'd serve ourselves. A huge part of losing 10 pounds is learning to identify a smart portion when dining out. Always opt for the smallest portion size available. Many restaurants offer a "bistro size" or "lunch portion" of their salads and entrées. This portion size will leave you happy and full at 99 percent of restaurants. Or, order an appetizer version of a full entrée, such a veggie quesadilla or steamed mussels. When you find yourself wondering, "Will the half salad be enough?" remember that restaurants very often inflate portion sizes in order to charge more. Cut calories (and save money) by opting for the smaller portion.

After you eat, busy yourself with dishes and cleaning up your cooking space — this gives your brain a chance to register that your body is full, and you won't feel the need to grab another dinner roll or helping of potatoes.

Exercise nut portion control!

While studies have shown that people who include nuts in their diets often have lower risk of heart disease, nuts are also very calorie-dense, much of which is from fat. Nuts are only beneficial if they are eaten in careful moderation and do not significantly contribute to your daily calorie count. Unfortunately, because nuts come in large tins and bags, it is just too easy to snack on them by the handful and wreak havoc on your weight loss.

Know that not all nuts are created equal! Good nuts include almonds, walnuts, peanuts and pistachios. Not-so-good nuts, such as macadamias, pecans and Brazil nuts, are high in fat and calories. Because all nuts are calorie-dense, stick to about an ounce of nuts, which equals 160 to 200 calories.

NutHealth.org lists the following as the number of nuts per serving:

Extremeness aversion is the tendency to avoid the smallest and largest sizes and order the middle size — no matter how large. Be wary of this when you order items like movie theater popcorn and soda at fast-food restaurants, and always stick to the smallest size.

- Almonds: 20-24
- Cashews: 16-18
- Macadamias: 10-12
- Brazil nuts: 6-8
- Hazelnuts: 18-20
- Pecans: 18-20 halves
- Pistachios: 45-47
- Pine Nuts: 150-157
- Walnuts: 8-11 halves

Nuts make an easy, crunchy snack, just make sure you always count them out into snack-size baggies. Never try to ration while eating from a jar or bag of nuts — you'll surely overdo it. And be smart: Pass on anything honey-roasted, candied, oil-roasted, or covered in chocolate or yogurt. Raw, unsalted, unroasted nuts are the ones that will make you feel full and satisfied while keeping your calories down. In the right portions, they can be part of a successful weight-loss plan.

Ask for a doggie bag right away

Another smart dieters' trick is to ask for a doggie bag or to-go container as soon as your entrée touches down on the table. Determine an appropriate portion and set aside the rest for leftovers. When the entire meal stays on your plate, you are constantly tempted to keep eating and eating until your plate is bare. Think about how many times you've thought, *Well, I've eaten two-thirds of this meal already, so I may as well finish the rest.* Store half your meal out of sight and feel content when the plate is empty.

Split your meal in half

You can cut calories and still enjoy your favorite foods by dividing your meal and only eating half. One way to do this is to split your meal with a friend. Or, if you and your dining companion can't agree, you can substitute the other half of your meal with a broth-based soup, fresh veggies, or a piece of fruit. For instance, instead of two slices of pepperoni pizza, replace the second piece of pizza with a garden salad and light dressing. This simple change can save you about 350 calories. Substitute water with lemon or sparkling water, like Perrier, instead of a soda and you've saved 500 calories right there.

❝Divide each difficulty into as many parts as is feasible and necessary to resolve it. **❞**

~ Rene Descartes

Chapter 6

Put an End to Mindless Eating

With our busy lives and schedules, so much of eating happens while we multitask or are on-the-go — at desks, in front of the TV, with friends, or in cars. Unfortunately, eating while distracted or while working on something else at the same time leads to overeating. Mindless eating is the downfall of many dieters. The hand-to-mouth action of eating can become addictive and, before you know it, you've gone through a large bag of chips or eaten an entire plate of fries that you didn't even order! Losing weight comes from holding yourself accountable — including your guilty pleasures, little indulgences and bad habits.

You must learn to pay attention while food is around you. One key is, of course, keeping a food diary, which is the single-best way to stay accountable for and aware of what you're eating. Stop functioning on auto-pilot and start paying attention to what you're eating, when you're eating, and where you're eating. Most environments offer cues and clues that you may be tempted to eat too much, and you must pay attention to those and get your willpower ready. You probably also harbor several unconscious habits that cause you to snack and eat without even realizing it. These are opportunities to change your behavior and cut hundreds of extra calories from your day!

Because food provides pleasure and comfort for so many people, and because calories sneak up on you in so many places, you must stop mindlessly eating in order to lose up to 10 pounds in 2 weeks. Wake up! Pay attention! Savor the healthy foods you eat but make eating an experience more about fueling your body than about enjoyment. Truly, the most wonderful feeling will be when you step on the scale at the end of each week and see the weight dropping off!

Just like the old adage, "Don't grocery shop while you're hungry," don't cook while you're starving either. Start making a meal before you're hungry so you don't snack while cooking.

Keep a food diary!

A hugely important step to eating fewer calories and burning through unwanted pounds is keeping a food diary. Keeping track of what you eat and drink keeps you accountable and aware and prevents mindless snacking. Luckily, this journal comes equipped with a 14-day food and fitness diary, but you'll want to keep maintaining one even after you've lost your 10 pounds. Why? For one, you probably have no idea how many calories or grams of fat are in much of what you eat. Research has shown again and again that people grossly underestimate the number of calories in their food — they are usually off by about 50 percent! Additionally, people tend to have generous and selective memories when it comes to what they have eaten. How many times have you "forgotten" about a half of a muffin, a handful of crackers, or finishing your child's cookie?

A study in the *American Journal of Preventive Medicine* followed 1,700 overweight or obese men and women (the average weight was 212 pounds) who were following an exercise and diet plan. The subjects who did not record what they ate lost 9 pounds. However, those who did keep a food journal lost twice as much weight, or an average of 18 pounds. So keep your food and fitness journal up-to-date and be accountable for every bite and sip!

Are you a snacking chef?

Are you constantly "taste testing" your chili every few minutes? Do you snack on shredded cheese while you're dicing taco toppings? Does licking the egg beaters after making a dessert date back to a childhood habit? What's the point of preparing a healthy meal for yourself or your family if you're snacking the whole time, adding hundreds of extra calories? Just like the old adage, "Don't grocery shop while you're hungry," don't cook while you're starving either. Start making a meal before you're hungry so the food is ready by the time you're eager to eat. If it's too late and you're already hungry, set aside a small plate of veggies, such as carrots or crunchy cucumber slices, to enjoy while you cook. A spoonful of peanut butter or a few crackers can also hold you over for a while so you aren't tempted to lick the bowl after making banana bread. Start paying attention when you cook and don't let hundreds of needless calories sneak in.

Beware of drive-by snacking

Food is often presented in a way that makes it seem casual, easy and friendly a bowl of M&M's on someone's desk at work, kiosks of samples at Costco, attractive hors d'oeuvres at a party, or a tray of bite-size tasters at the coffee shop. Without thinking, you grab a handful of candy each time you walk to your cubicle. At a party, you take something off every tray of hors d'oeuvres that comes around. As you chat with friends, "Ooh, I'll try that," becomes, "Sure, I'll have another." Soon you have a pile of cocktail napkins and crumbs in your hand. People often get the misperception that a few bites here and a few bites there are OK — but they add up quickly. You must eliminate drive-by snacking if you're going to cut out the hundreds of calories you need to reach your goal of 10 pounds in 2 weeks. Avoid opportunities for mindless snacking. Don't spend a long time chatting with a coworker who has candy or cookies at his or her desk, but if you must, be mindful of the presence of temptation and don't give in!

Did You Know?

How many food-related choices do you think you make in a day? When a Cornell University team of researchers posed this question to participants, the average answer was 14. However, when the participants were asked to more closely consider a typical day, it showed that they actually made an average of 226 food decisions a day. One author of the study concluded: "... It is not unfair to say we often engage in mindless eating."

Look out for liquid calories!

Are you drinking your calories? Juice, smoothies, sweetened tea, sports drinks, energy drinks, protein shakes, and alcohol are all packed with calories, sugar and carbs, just like soda, and sometimes more so. Plus, have you ever looked closely at the labels of your Gatorade, Naked Juice, Arizona Iced Tea or Monster? Most bottled drinks contain more than 1 serving — 2.5 servings per bottle is typical. If you drink the whole bottle, which most people do, you're drinking 200 to 400 calories in just a few gulps. The real problem is that liquids don't fill you up, so you wind up eating on top of what you're drinking. Satiation comes from chewing, thus many times a liquid will be ingested unconsciously in just a few gulps, without helping you to feel full and without any thought for the calories you just consumed. It's easy to forget about 250 calories when they're in liquid form, but cutting out 250 calories can make a big difference in the amount of weight you lose. Drinks are a quick and easy place to cut extra calories to lose more weight.

Are you drinking your calories? Juice, smoothies, sweetened tea, sports drinks, energy drinks, protein shakes, and alcohol are all packed with calories, sugar and carbs, just like soda, and sometimes more so.

Beware of bite-size

Unfortunately, our brains often trick us into thinking that eating something bite-size means it's better for us than eating the same food in its full size. But this is only true if you eat just a few bite-size pieces! And studies have shown that small treats, such as mini-cookies, actually lead people to eat more than they would if the cookies were full-size. If you wouldn't eat a whole cheese Danish, why eat four samples at the coffee shop? You're not doing your waistline any favors, and you're actually doing yourself a double disservice by pretending those calories don't count. Whenever samples of high-calorie treats are nearby, such as pastries at a coffee shop, remind yourself that even small bites add up to hundreds of calories.

Be the life of the party without overindulging

Always eat consciously. At a party, be wary of the hand-to-mouth motion while you're chatting with friends. You don't need to accept every time a waiter comes by offering hors d'oeuvre. Hors d'oeuvres are always rich and fatty in order to pack lots of flavor in a small bite. Items like filled puff pastries, crab cakes, deviled eggs, bacon-wrapped shrimp, and creamy dips are popular and each has a ton of calories. You could be consuming 100 calories or more per bite! When you attend an event or party, stand away from the entrance to the kitchen so you're not the first guest servers with hot, fresh trays of hors d'oeuvres see. Also, a great calorie-saving trick for parties is to fill up lighter fare, such as crunchy crudités (raw veggies), shrimp cocktail, or smoked salmon, and allow yourself only one indulgent treat. Eat one bite to be sure it's truly delicious and worth the calories. If it's not, toss the rest away.

A study in the journal Obesity reported that people consume an average of 236 more calories on Saturdays than on any other day of the week.

Never eat in front of the TV

More than 66 percent of Americans report that they regularly watch TV while dining at home. Unfortunately, people who watch television while eating tend to overeat without being aware of it. Studies have shown that people can eat almost an entire extra meal's worth of calories on days when they eat in front of the TV. Television distracts you from responding naturally to your body's cues of hunger and fullness. Turning on the TV can trigger the desire to snack even if you are not hungry. You also tend to rely on external cues, such as the end of a show, rather than internal cues to stop eating. Keep the TV off and sit down at the table to savor the flavor, color, and texture of your food. You'll eat hundreds fewer calories than you would zoning out on the couch.

Keep food far from your bedside

Having food in bed is a habit that dates back to childhood for many people. You may have enjoyed a warm glass of milk in bed in order to have a better night of sleep. Maybe your mother brought you soup in bed when you weren't feeling well. Or perhaps the concept of "breakfast in bed" was seen as an indulgence meant for Dad on Father's Day. Whatever the case may be, know that eating in bed only promotes mindless eating. Bringing a bag of popcorn or a tub of ice cream into bed while you watch a movie or curl up with a book is simply setting the stage for overeating (not to mention making a mess!). Again, practice conscious eating by keeping food in the setting in which it belongs — at the dinner table.

Look out for overeating cues

Environments that lead to overeating tend to give you cues and clues that too much food is on its way — now you just have to pay attention to them! Family style serving dishes, heaping bread baskets, short and wide drink glasses, carafes of soda or wine, buffet-style presentation, and oversized pasta and salad bowls are simply putting the temptation to grossly overeat in front of you. It's not just restaurants that are the culprit either; take a look around your own home for these items as well. Make your home less conducive to overeating and stay better aware of portion control.

> Pay attention to environmental cues and clues that too much food is on its way. Family style serving dishes, carafes of soda or wine, buffet-style presentation, and oversized pasta and salad bowls are simply putting the temptation to grossly overeat in front of you.

In a portion of the Cornell Food and Brand Lab study "Mindless Eating: The 200 Daily Food Decisions We Overlook," researchers measured the amount eaten by 379 participants, half of whom were served with a particularly large bowl or plate of food. The participants given the extra-large servings ate an average of 31 percent more food than the participants with the normal-sized dinnerware. More interestingly, even when researchers later revealed to those participants that they had been given an extra-large portion, 21 percent denied having eaten more, 75 percent attributed it to other reasons (such as hunger), and only 4 percent attributed it to the environmental cue of the oversized plate or bowl. Researchers concluded that we are either unaware of how our environment influences eating decisions or we are unwilling to acknowledge it.

Don't be one of the many people who is biased by the size of packaging, presentation, and plating. Look for common cues and clues and either stay away from environments that offer the temptation to overeat or be so conscious of the temptation that you monitor your intake carefully.

Make your own 100-calorie snack packs

Never snack on things like popcorn, nuts, dried fruit or crackers straight from the bag or package; you'll definitely overdo it. Bags and boxes of snack foods make it difficult to determine a proper portion size. Instead, make your own 100-calorie snack packs so you'll never be without a healthy, low-calorie snack. Put baby carrots, celery sticks, almonds, dried apricots, and whole wheat crackers into small baggies and have them in your purse, desk, backpack or wherever you'll need them.

TV can trigger the desire to snack, and you tend to rely on external cues, such as the end of a show, rather than internal cues to stop eating. Keep the TV off and sit down at the table to savor your food.

While 100-calorie packs of treats, such as cookies, chips and candy, are now available, you should only purchase those tempting, sugary or salty snacks if you know you have the willpower to eat just one package. If chocolate chip cookies or potato chips are a trigger food for you, 100-calorie packs are just needless temptation.

Beware of Saturday diet sabotage

A study in the journal *Obesity* reported that people consume an average of 236 more calories on Saturdays than on any other day of the week. Theories on why? For one, your weekends aren't as structured as weekdays, where you have set times for lunch breaks, dinner, etc. Thus, people tend to eat carelessly and at odd times. Also, people tend to the view the weekend as time to relax and take a break from the routine of the workweek, thus, they tend to turn their backs on their diets and seriously overeat. However, losing up to 10 pounds in 2 weeks requires structure, and not just Monday through Friday. Don't let a lazy Saturday lead you to indulge in a calorie-rich meal. If you want to think of Saturday as a day to take it easy, use it as one of your days off from working out. But that's all the more reason to pass on a fatty meal!

Hors d'oeuvres are always rich in order to pack flavor in a small bite. Items like filled puff pastries, crab cakes, deviled eggs, bacon-wrapped shrimp, and creamy dips can have 100 calories or more per bite!

❝ Let us not be content to wait and see what will happen, but give us the determination to make the right things happen. **❞**

~ Horace Mann

Chapter 7

No More Emotional Eating

Ever heard of eating your feelings? Emotional eating is a huge problem for overweight people and in most failed diets, because the very nature of being overweight causes stress, anxiety, sadness and loneliness, which all contribute to the cycle of emotional eating. A study published in the journal *Obesity* reported that people who practice emotional eating have a much harder time losing weight, and those who do lose weight are more likely to regain it. The study concluded that, to be truly successful, weight-loss programs needed to teach their clients coping skills to replace emotional eating practices.

Emotional eating is simply a coping strategy. Anything from relationship problems to unemployment to depression to work-related stress can lead to emotional eating. Many times, emotional eating habits are ingrained and reinforced in us over the years, as we get older and the responsibilities and stresses increase with adulthood. And, unfortunately, emotional eaters are typically only interested in fatty or sugary snacks that completely derail their diet plans.

As this chapter reveals, positive emotions and people you love may be causing you to emotionally eat as well. You'll learn to recognize the triggers that lead you to overeat out of celebration, or the friends and loved ones who mean well but are actually wreaking havoc on your weight.

This chapter reveals fascinating facts about how eating in a social setting, with your significant other or family members, or around coworkers can determine how much and what you eat. You'll also learn about how your gender affects your calorie intake.

In reality, emotional eating revolves around having a very unhealthy relationship with food — using it as a coping mechanism, a comfort, a distraction from your problems, a means to fit in, or a reward. And when emotional eating spirals out of control, it becomes binge eating, the most common form of disordered eating, which affects approximately 2 million Americans, according to the National Institute of Mental Health. Binge eating disorder, like emotional eating, involves uncontrollable, excessive eating, followed by feelings of shame and guilt.

Whether you're overeating in a group of friends or pigging out on late-night junk food when you're home alone, you need to confront your bad habits and find better ways to cope with emotional changes and disruptions. Because emotional eating habits are some of the most difficult to change (they often date back decades to childhood), these are also the behaviors that frustrate people and keep them from losing significant weight.

Feeling powerless to food and your weight is a daily struggle. But learning the emotional triggers, people and situations that lead you to make unhealthy choices is the only way to break the nasty cycle of overeating that causes sadness and anxiety and, in turn, more overeating. Wouldn't you love to feel in control of your eating habits for once in your life? Wouldn't you love to find other, healthy ways to address stress, conflict, personal issues or to celebrate, without ruining your weight-loss efforts? Read on to figure out how to eat for nutrition and lose weight rather than feeding your feelings.

Recognize that emotional eating makes you feel worse

Emotional eating is a horrible cycle because it both stems from and creates feelings of sadness, stress and embarrassment. How many times have you heard someone say: "I eat because I'm sad, and then I'm sad because I'm fat"? People will binge on ice cream or alcohol when they feel sad, and then, in turn, feel much worse after realizing how many empty calories they just ingested. And the more overweight people get, the more they isolate themselves and soothe themselves with food.

Because emotional eating habits are some of the most difficult to change (they often date back decades to childhood), these are also the behaviors that frustrate people and keep them from losing significant weight.

As David L. Katz, M.D., a professor of public health and medicine at Yale University School of Medicine, says, "You can't make food the solution to every issue in your life and expect to be thin." Stop burying your thin, happy self under high-calorie meals! Your goal of losing up to 10 pounds in 2 weeks can be met with awareness, willpower and dedication. Once you realize how much better you feel from eating healthy and losing weight, you'll never want to fall into the cycle of emotional eating again.

Recognize these amazing differences between emotional hunger and physical hunger

You must learn the differences between and recognize the cues of emotional and physical hunger to find ways to deal with cravings and avoid overeating. There are several ways to tell whether what you're experiencing is true, internal hunger or whether your body and mind are responding to external emotions. Emotional hunger comes on suddenly, out of nowhere, and is associated with an event or emotion, such as having a fight with your spouse. Physical hunger is gradual; it comes on slowly and includes physical cues, such as a grumbling stomach, hunger pains, or slight fatigue. Emotional eating is typically for a specific food — chocolate or a cheeseburger — and needs to be satisfied immediately. Real, physical hunger can wait several minutes or even hours and a wide range of foods will satisfy it. Emotional hunger is not really related to fullness, so you may eat very quickly and won't stop eating when you feel full. You may also feel distracted and find that you eat a whole bag of chips or box of cookies without realizing it. Physical hunger, however, responds to fullness, and you will stop eating when you're satisfied. Likewise, you eat consciously and slowly, enjoying your food. Emotional hunger is coupled with feelings of guilt and shame for overeating, whereas physical hunger is not accompanied by negative feelings. With physical hunger, you recognize food as fuel and eating a necessary part of your day. Finally, emotional hunger may come on soon after you've already eaten. If you feel a craving coming on an hour or two after your last meal or snack, you can bet it's probably not true, physical hunger. With these differences in mind, you should be able to determine which type of hunger you're experiencing. If it's not physical

Did You Know?

How common is emotional eating? Emotional eating may be a factor in as much as 75 percent of all overeating, according to the Department of Nutrition Therapy at the Cleveland Clinic.

hunger, focus on putting a stop to the craving instead of indulging it.

Head off emotional eating at the pass

Eating out of emotion is what is a called a "negative coping pattern," meaning that you are simply compounding your problems by being overweight. Awareness means stopping emotional eating before it starts. Figure out which types of bad feelings and situations lead you to eat out of emotion, rather than hunger. The five most typical emotions or states that cause overeating are loneliness, boredom, anger, stress, and fatigue. If your hand ends up in the bottom of the Snackwells after a fight with your sister, make a mental note of it. If your first reaction to an extra-stressful day at work is to stop for a cheeseburger and 6-pack of beer on the way home, be aware of that negative coping pattern. Then you will be able to anticipate and stop emotional eating down the road.

> Emotional hunger is coupled with feelings of guilt and shame for overeating, whereas physical hunger is not accompanied by negative feelings. With physical hunger, you recognize food as fuel and eating a necessary part of your day.

Remove temptation!

It sounds basic, but if you don't have trigger foods around the house, you'll have fewer opportunities to overeat. You know the kinds of snacks and desserts you crave late at night, when you're watching a movie, or when you've had a bad day. Now, make a list of the things you can have instead — a 100-calorie serving of popcorn, raw veggies, a low-fat yogurt, or low-sugar cereal.

Find other outlets for celebration or comfort

You got fired, you got a promotion, you broke up with your boyfriend, your team won the Super Bowl — so you eat half a pizza. You tell yourself, "I deserve this." You use food to both celebrate and to help you lick your wounds. But what sense does it make to let circumstances largely out of your control so greatly affect your diet and weight? Why would you want the glow of new job to be outshined by the guilt you feel for eating a pound of Buffalo wings at your celebratory happy hour? Don't use food as comfort or celebration. Find other ways to give yourself a pat on the back or relieve anger and stress during a trying time. Had a great day? Go shopping and treat yourself to a new pair of shoes. Do something that makes you feel great, other than overindulging in food, like getting a massage. Had a crappy day? Need a shoulder to cry on? A burrito isn't going to provide the emotional support you need. Call a friend instead. Or sweat it out at the gym. Exercise is the number one stress reliever. And obviously, when you're exercising you're doing something beneficial for your body, as opposed to indulging in a calorie-packed meal.

Recognize if a friend or loved one is sabotaging your weight loss

While it is natural to expect that the ones who care for you would want to support you in your efforts to lose weight, many people find that certain friends and family members actually sabotage their weight loss — intentionally and unintentionally. Take a look at the person in question — typically, he or she is also struggling with weight, overeating and a sedentary lifestyle. Some people feel better about their unhealthy lifestyle choices when you live the same way. Many times, the person you are closest to has long been your partner in crime when it comes to unhealthy eating. He or she will feel isolated and jealous when you start making better food choices and pass on the beer-and-pizza-Saturdays that have become your tradition. Explain to this person that losing weight and keeping it off is going to require a complete lifestyle makeover, and you want and need his or her love and support to be successful.

Stop the late-night snack attack

Dieticians and nutritionists commonly say that late-night eating is their clients' biggest problem that keeps them from losing weight. They eat smart all day only to fall victim to midnight munchies. Does that sound like you? Learn to ward of the late-night snack attack by determining why you're tempted to eat so late. There is an off-chance that you've restricted your calories so much throughout the day, and so you're actually hungry before bed. If so, try adding more fiber or protein to your dinner to feel fuller longer.

But truly, late-night snacking is just another form of emotional eating. Loneliness, boredom and stress are three of the most typical emotions that cause eating for reasons other than hunger, especially when you're home late at night. To avoid eating out of the desire for comfort or to relax, look for other things to fulfill this need, such as a bath or exchanging massages with your spouse. If you know you're going to be unwinding at home, find something to do with your hands other than eating, such as drinking a mug of tea. Warm liquids are also said to have a calming and de-stressing effect that

While it is natural to expect that the ones who care for you would want to support you in your efforts to lose weight, many people find that certain friends and family members actually sabotage their weight loss — intentionally and unintentionally.

helps get ready for a good night of sleep. Or, find an activity that includes both hands so you won't have one hand on your book and the other in a bag of Doritos. Type an email to a friend or knit. Cleaning can also be a good stress reliever that keeps you busy and out of the fridge. Whatever it takes, tell yourself you're done eating for the night after you have a healthy dinner.

Don't eat more in the company of others — male or female

A 2009 study in the journal *Appetite* studied the effects of eating in social settings on both men and women an discovered that women who ate in all female groups ate significantly more than if they ate alone, on a date, or in a group that included men. When men were at the table, the women ate about 450 calories each. By contrast, in an all-female group, the number rose to about 750 calories. Interestingly, while men were not affected by the gender of their company, they consumed more than 700 calories per meal regardless, which was higher than all the women in the study.

Maintain your willpower when eating with friends! A study showed that when men were at the table, a group of women ate about 450 calories each. By contrast, in an all-female group, the number rose to about 750 calories.

The bottom line is, social environments lead to poor impulse control and overeating. Surely you've heard the phrase "Eat, drink and be merry." If your mindset is that eating out with friends is an indulgence or treat, you're more likely to indulge in high-calorie food, desserts and drinks. Both sexes should feel confident enough to say "No thanks" when a dinner companion suggests splitting the fried calamari or cheesecake. Alcohol and coffee drinks also rack up major calories, so order hot tea if everyone is having after-dinner drinks. Or suggest social activities that don't include eating! Do something exercise-related, such as arranging for a group bike ride, hike or entering a 5k with friends.

Know the few times when it's OK to give in

Certain holidays and special occasions, such as a birthday, Thanksgiving, family reunion, or New Year's Eve, mean you will want to indulge in a rich dessert, buttery mashed potatoes or a few glasses of champagne — and you have to know that it's OK to do so. Treating yourself, rarely and only when the occasion is particularly meaningful, shows a healthy and well-balanced approach to eating. You're not using to food to celebrate,

The five most typical emotions or states that cause overeating are loneliness, boredom, anger, stress, and fatigue.

per se, but you're enjoying a special moment with loved ones that includes a dietary indulgence. Just plan ahead. If you know you're going to spend a few hundred calories on these treats, you need to plan throughout the day and week to cut back in other areas.

" Develop success from failures. Discouragement and failure are two of the surest stepping stones to success. **"**

~ Dale Carnegie

Chapter 8

Choosing Healthy Alternatives

Americans tend to run in the other direction when they hear the word "healthy." Indeed, many people mistakenly believe that foods that are healthy are unsatisfying or taste bad. In a new *Journal of Consumer Research* study, researchers found that when people were asked to taste food described as "healthy," they reported being hungrier afterward than those who ate the same food when it was described as "tasty." In one portion of the study, some students were told they were sampling a new protein-, vitamin- and fiber-packed "health bar"; others were told it was a "chocolate bar that is very tasty and yummy with a chocolate-raspberry core." When they were later asked to rate their hunger, those who sampled the "health bar" rated themselves hungrier than those who ate the identical "tasty" bar. In a second portion of the study, participants were given a piece of bread either described as being "low-fat and nutritious" or "tasty, with a thick crust and soft center." After sampling the bread, participants were offered pretzels; those who ate the "healthy" bread ate more pretzels than those who sampled the "tasty" bread. This study showed that not only do people expect healthy food to be unsatisfying, it actually makes them hungrier than if they had eaten nothing at all. In the end, "healthy" foods made subjects eat in excess.

As a nation, we have been somewhat brainwashed to view reduced or low-fat foods as second-class to the original. But in many cases, reduced fat or low-cal foods are indistinguishable from their higher calorie counterparts. Sometimes, the low-fat version is actually tastier! To lose up to 10 pounds in 2 weeks, you need to change your perception that healthy foods will not satisfy you as much as your favorite dishes. In fact, you will probably find that once you continuously substitute vegetables, fruits and whole grains for greasy, fried fast-food meals, you will start to prefer the fresh, clean taste of lower-calorie foods.

Half of a large grapefruit has 50 calories, 2 grams of fiber, and 11 grams of sugar while 8 fluid ounces of grapefruit juice contains about 100 calories and 22 grams of sugar. When you're craving something sweet and juicy, reach for the real piece of fruit rather than juice.

In order to lose weight, you must make healthy tradeoffs. Giving up desserts in favor of fruit, for instance, can help you drop unwanted pounds quickly. Or eating out less and cooking at home more — although eating out may be more fun — saves hundreds of calories at each meal. In weight loss, tradeoffs usually mean giving up something you enjoy for something less instantly gratifying but healthier in the long run. Diet tradeoffs are worth it because reaching an ideal weight, feeling great and being healthier are the ultimate payoffs.

Nothing will be more motivating than recognizing bad habits, beginning new ones, and seeing the unwanted pounds come off! Mark Twain once joked, "The only way to keep your health is to eat what you don't want,

Stay Motivated!
"Optimism is the faith that leads to achievement.
Nothing can be done without hope and confidence."
~ Helen Keller

drink what you don't like, and do what you'd rather not." But this doesn't have to be true! Being healthy and losing 10 pounds is really all about making smart tradeoffs that have real benefits to you.

Modify recipes with healthy ingredient substitutions

There's no need to toss out your favorite recipes — just find healthy substitutions for the high-calorie ingredients. Your favorite dishes will retain their flavor and save you hundreds of calories. You won't even notice the difference! A favorite diet secret is substituting Greek or other non-fat yogurt for sour cream and mayo. You won't lose any of the creaminess but with zero grams of fat and packed with protein, you're making a smart tradeoff. Tofu is also good substitute for many ingredients because it is rich in high-quality protein and contains no cholesterol. Try using it in place of cream in sauces. Replace ground beef with lean ground chicken or turkey. If a vegetable recipe calls for butter or margarine, use chicken broth and herbs for flavor without the fat. Replace whole eggs with two egg whites and just a tiny bit of yolk. Use condensed skim milk for whole milk. Replace the sugar in baking recipes with the no-calorie sweetener Splenda.

Choose the right salad dressings

Salads can, of course, be one of your best weight-loss friends. Frequently eating green salads with raw veggies means your body will be getting crucial nutrients and antioxidants, such as vitamins A, C and E, folic acid, fiber, lycopene, and beta-carotene. However, to lose up to 10 pounds in 2 weeks, you need to be consider the dressings you're choosing. A study of 1,000 people by Kraft Foods found that the top choices of salad dressing for women were Ranch, blue cheese and vinaigrette. Men's top choices were Ranch, blue cheese, and French/Catalina, and Thousand Island. Clearly, creamy dressings are the favorites of both men and women. They are also the quickest way to turn your healthy meal into salad sabotage. And, beware of vinaigrettes that load up with sugar to achieve better taste.

To save hundreds of calories and dozens of grams of fat, ask for oil and vinegar. A few splashes of red wine or balsamic vinegar are often all you need on a vegetable salad. Even better? Squeeze a fresh lemon over your salad for a zero-calorie dressing. If you can't live without your favorite dressings, many, such as Caesar and Raspberry Vinaigrette, come in a spray bottle version with only 1 calorie per spray (10 sprays are enough for a 1-cup salad). Don't turn your healthy salad into a 1,000-calorie nightmare; choose the right dressings.

Did You Know?

Data from the National Health and Nutrition Examination Survey compared fruit and vegetable intake to USDA recommendations. Shockingly, less than 1% of adolescents, about 2% of men, and only 3.5% of women met guidelines for both fruits and vegetables — despite counting foods like jelly and orange juice as fruit, and both French fries and ketchup as vegetables. Eat more fruits and veggies!

Cook veggies the right way!

Never cook vegetables with butter, excessive oil, cream or in the deep fryer. Instead, try a splash of lemon juice, a drizzle of balsamic vinegar or a twist of black pepper before oven-baking vegetables like cauliflower or sweet potatoes. Leave out the pads of butter from recipes like curried carrots — the rich spices already give the carrots a great flavor without the added calories and saturated fat. Experiment and you'll find that many vegetables, like tomatoes and bell peppers, are delicious when baked or blackened on a grill, without adding much of anything. Remember, the fewer ingredients the better when it comes to keeping vegetables low-fat and low-calorie.

Have whole fruits instead of juices

Whole fruits can help you lose weight because they contain essential phytonutrients and their fiber and water content help you feel satisfied. On the flip side, commercial fruit juice usually includes added sugars and 100 or more calories per glass. Also, when the pulp and skin of the fruit is removed, the sugar absorbs quickly within the body and can cause cravings later in the day. Juicing removes the bulk of the fruit so juice does not fill you up like the real fruit does. Half of a large grapefruit has 50 calories, 2 grams of fiber, and 11 grams of sugar while 8 fluid ounces of grapefruit juice contains about 100 calories and 22 grams of sugar. When you're craving something sweet and juicy, reach for the real piece of fruit rather than sugary juice. For a dessert substitute, try putting pineapple slices or halved peaches on the grill for a warm, sweet treat without high fructose corn syrup and added calories.

> To save hundreds of calories and dozens of grams of fat, ask for oil and vinegar. A few splashes of red wine or balsamic vinegar are often all you need on a vegetable salad. Even better? Squeeze a fresh lemon over your salad for a zero-calorie dressing.

Pass on ready-made grocery store salads

When you're cutting calories, pass on ready-made grocery store salads from the deli aisle. Typical choices — English pea, pasta, potato, Waldorf, macaroni, broccoli, chicken, tuna and egg salads — are all full of mayo. It's

A favorite diet secret is substituting Greek or other non-fat yogurt for sour cream and mayo. You won't lose any of the creaminess but with zero grams of fat and packed with protein, you're making a smart tradeoff.

what holds these salads together, giving them their consistency. These are not healthy sides. These are not "salads" like you want them to be — "salads" meaning fresh, healthy and satisfying. A better choice that you can make on your own in a hurry: fruit salad. Chop a banana, apple and red grapes and add a can of drained mandarin oranges. Sprinkle cinnamon over the top and you have enough to feed two to four people a sweet side salad with no fat and only natural sugars. Another healthier, lighter option is to make tuna salad Mediterranean style, with chopped celery, olives, olive oil, lemon juice, and salt and pepper.

Enjoy a delicious bowl of soup

Warm liquids not only help calm and relax the body, they provide a sense of satiation because they must be ingested slowly. Thus, vegetable soup is a great weight-loss food. Soup is relatively low in calories per serving, and the high water content sends messages to your brain that you're full. You'll have to slow down while eating the hot soup and bites are always a spoonful. Have a tomato-based soup with high-fiber whole grains, beans, vegetables, and/or lean meat. If the bowl is small, pair it with a turkey sandwich on whole wheat bread (hold the mayo to eliminate extra calories). The extra ingredients will take time to digest and leave you feeling full longer. Avoid cream-based soups since they contain butter and fat and are high in calories.

Incorporate veggies in unexpected ways

Not everyone who wants to lose weight also enjoys eating vegetables.

Even people who love veggies typically don't eat enough of them! Rather than sitting down with a pile of produce and forcing yourself to eat it, try sneaking vegetables into dishes you already love. You won't even notice they're there, and you'll be getting the nutrients and fiber you need to lose weight and stay healthy. Some great ideas for incorporating vegetables in unexpected ways include pureeing carrots and zucchini in marinara sauce, meatballs, and burger patties; adding sweet potatoes to pancake batter; substituting baked butternut squash for pasta in mac 'n' cheese; and using steamed cauliflower in mashed potatoes. Vegetables are a crucial part of losing weight, because they are fiber-dense but low in calories, so they fill you up longer for fewer calories. Plus, veggies are packed with natural minerals and vitamins to ward off illness and disease. Just because you're a former steak-and-potatoes type or you're trying to cook for a family that refuses to eat their vegetables, doesn't mean you can't get the nutrients and fiber your body craves to lose weight.

Satisfy a sweet tooth with spices

There are many ways you can satisfy a sweet tooth without cookies, cakes, candy, or ice cream. The urge for something sweet can often be satisfied when you add spices to certain foods. Add the spices commonly found in desserts — vanilla, cinnamon, nutmeg, clove, ginger, and allspice — to other foods that are already naturally sweet, such as baked apples, pears, peaches and sweet potatoes. You can achieve the flavors and sweetness you crave from baked goods without all the extra sugar, fat, and calories.

Warm liquids not only help calm and relax the body, they provide a sense of satiation because they must be ingested slowly. Thus, vegetable soup is a great weight-loss food.

Find a low-calorie alternative to your daily latte

Unless you specify, coffee drinks are made with 2% milk, which adds fat, calories and carbs to your beverage. Additionally, any sweetener, such as flavored syrups, caramel, or cocoa powder, add dozens of calories and carbs as well. And specialty drinks typically include whipped cream, chocolate shavings and other high-calorie toppings. Even if you opt for a light or "skinny" version of your favorite latte, you're looking at 200 calories.

If you can't live without coffee, the key to losing weight is to go as pared down as possible with your selections. Start with hot or iced Café Americano (aka, regular coffee). Sounds dull? It doesn't have to be! One or two pumps of sugar-free flavored syrup can jazz it up. A splash of nonfat milk is reasonable. Cinnamon is also a favorite coffee condiment of many dieters. It packs lots of flavor without the added sugar. Making this switch will let you start your day with under 25 calories per medium coffee, creating a 100-calorie-plus deficit, right from the start of your day.

Don't dip into fat and calories

Trim Up to 300 Calories!

Pass: Granola with raisins, or
Swap: Turkey pepperoni instead of salami pepperoni

Dips are popular at barbecues, potlucks and housewarming parties, but most — spinach and artichoke, French onion, 7-layer bean dip — are jam-packed with fat and calories in every spoonful. Most of the most popular party dips are the creamy and cheesy versions, which have 200 calories or more per ¼-cup serving, more than 10 grams of fat, and include several grams of saturated fat.

If you're attending or hosting a party, skip the veggie tray from the grocery store, which almost always includes Ranch dressing. Buy veggies individually (usually cheaper than the pre-made tray anyhow), such as grape tomatoes, celery sticks, bell peppers, cauliflower and snap peas, and make your own healthy dip. A great one, even for the cooking-challenged, is hummus, which is just chickpeas, olive oil, tahini, lemon juice, garlic, and black and cayenne pepper blended to a smooth texture in a food processor. Or to make Mediterranean layered dip, a perfect substitute for high-calorie bean dip, you can stack low-fat Greek yogurt, kalamata olives, feta, tomatoes, red pepper, cucumbers, garlic and whatever else you like. Top it with chopped romaine lettuce and sprinkle paprika over the top for a healthy, hearty alternative.

Eat more natural peanut butter!

Natural peanut butter is a truly amazing diet food! It has heart-healthy monounsaturated fats and doesn't include the hydrogenated oils, sweeteners, and extra salt of other peanut butters. You'll notice the label on natural peanut butter includes only two ingredients: peanuts and salt. It's a great food for losing weight because it maintains blood sugar levels and has fiber to keep you feeling full longer. Instead of a high-calorie muffin for breakfast, eat two tablespoons of peanut butter on whole wheat toast. And peanut butter on a banana or apple is a great snack. Although it might have as many calories as a bag of chips, not all calories are created equal. Peanut butter's fiber and healthy fats keep you full longer so you'll eat less throughout the day.

All-natural peanut butter is a great food for losing weight because it maintains blood sugar levels and has fiber to keep you feeling full longer. Instead of a high-calorie muffin for breakfast, eat two tablespoons of peanut butter on whole wheat toast.

Don't mess up the most important meal of the day

Yes, you need to eat breakfast — but it's what you eat that is going to help you or keep you from losing 10 pounds. *Parade* magazine's annual report, "What America Really Eats," found that breakfast is actually becoming the highest calorie meal of the day for many people. That's because breakfast sandwiches and burritos — generally made with bacon, ham, cheese, fried potatoes and eggs made the top 10 on both men and women's lists of most-ordered menu items last year. Unfortunately, these items typically contain between 400 and 800 calories (not including the latte or orange juice you're probably washing them down with).

A better choice for weight loss? Protein-packed eggs. A study from the Pennington Biomedical Research Center showed that participants who ate two eggs for breakfast lost 65 percent more weight than participants who ate a bagel, even though the bagel and the eggs contained an equal number of calories. The egg-eaters also reported feeling more energetic than the participants who ate the bagels. Now, you do need some carbs, but make sure they're complex carbs such a whole wheat English muffin or oatmeal (without all the sugary toppings). Complex carbs make you feel full and burn directly into energy.

> A great weight-loss food? Protein-packed eggs. A study from the Pennington Biomedical Research Center showed that participants who ate two eggs for breakfast lost 65 percent more weight than participants who ate a bagel, even though the bagel and the eggs contained an equal number of calories.

Beware of low-fat products

A report called "Can Low Fat Nutrition Labels Lead to Obesity," published in the *Journal of Marketing Research*, offered a dose of reality as to why so many people don't lose a single pound from eating low-fat or fat-free foods. The study found that both normal-weight and overweight participants ate more when presented with a low-fat option of a nutrient-poor and calorie-rich snack food. Additionally, they found that overweight participants were more inclined than normal-weight people to overindulge. Why? The study contends that low-fat food labels increase consumption because they decrease guilt and give the false perception that you can eat more of the item. And it seemed that this was particularly true for overweight subjects.

Don't love veggies? Try sneaking them into dishes you already love. You won't even notice they're there, and you'll be getting the nutrients and fiber you need to lose weight and stay healthy.

In a portion of this study, a university open house and two gallon-size bowls of M&M's were set out, one labeled "New Colors of Regular M&M's" and the other labeled "New 'Low-Fat' M&M's" (although no such low-fat product currently exists). As expected, participants ate more M&M's (28.4 percent more!) when they were labeled as low fat than when they were labeled as regular. Furthermore, overweight participants took 16 percent more M&M's than normal-weight participants. While all participants increased their consumption, overweight subjects ate an average of 90 additional calories more of the candies labeled as "low fat."

❝ Never go backward. Attempt, and do it with all your might. **❞**

~ Charles Simmons

Chapter 9

What to Do When Dining Out

A recent survey found that the majority of dieters said that dining out represented the biggest challenge to their weight loss. While able to stick to their eating plan at home, at work, and even at friends' houses, once in a restaurant, their goals and willpower quickly unraveled. Why does dining out present such a challenge to so many people? One reason is that restaurant food is cooked primarily with your palate in mind, not your waistline. Indeed, chefs go to great lengths to include sauces, batters, and other calorie-laden accessories to dishes to improve their flavor and presentation.

Because you cannot control the meal's ingredients, you may end up eating far more calories than you would like. Statistics show that people eat an average of 500 calories more when dining out than at home. For example, if you made yourself a hamburger at home, you might choose a low-fat burger, or maybe even substitute it with a turkey or veggie burger. You might choose a low-fat or multi-grain bun, skip the cheese, and serve it with a small side salad. But in a restaurant, you will be served a giant burger, up to a half-pound in size. The burger could be topped with special sauces, cheese, and bacon and served with potato salad or fries on the side. Once these items are in front of you, you will surely be tempted to eat them.

To compound the problem, restaurant portions in the U.S. have nearly tripled in size over the last few decades. Have you ever heard someone who traveled abroad complain about the small portion sizes in Europe? That's because in Italy, for example, meat, pasta and vegetables are ordered and served as individual courses, whereas Americans are used to having all three come piled high in the same dish. In the U.S., you're eating far more at a restaurant than you would if you were cooking for yourself at home. A recent study showed that people consume 50 percent more calories, fat and sodium when they eat out. Therefore, when dining out you must make an extra effort to control the ingredients and portion size of the meal you order the same way you would when cooking at home. Don't be embarrassed to inquire about how something is prepared or served and ask for substitutions if necessary. And you never need to feel like you have to eat everything on your plate. The "clean plate" rule of your childhood no longer needs to apply!

Finally, as this chapter discusses, restaurant menus have been set up to make food sound as appealing as possible and many have photos, as well. The name of the Molten Chocolate Lava Cake with Crème Fraiche already sounds delicious, but when coupled with a photo, it's all you can do not to order one to enjoy all by yourself. And if the menu doesn't tempt you enough, the servers at restaurants have been coached to sell you certain dishes, drinks and desserts.

Luckily, American restaurants are finally beginning to accommodate the public's newfound interest in losing weight. National chains and fast-food restaurants now offer healthy or low-calorie dishes that help the calorie-conscious have a pleasant dining experience. And as part of the 2010 national health care reform bill, any fast-food or chain restaurant with 20 or more locations will be required to post calorie counts right on menus, menu boards and even drive-thrus. The idea is that with the nutritional information right in front of you, clueless eaters and calorie-counters alike will be able to make smart choices that eliminate hundreds of calories.

You never need to feel like you have to eat everything on your plate. The "clean plate" rule of your childhood no longer needs to apply!

Don't starve yourself all day before dining out

Don't make the common mistake of barely eating all day in anticipation of dinner with friends. You'll be starving come dinnertime and you'll overeat. Instead, eat normally throughout the day and have a small snack before you leave for your dinner. According to Purdue University research, eating a handful of peanuts about an hour before dinner will cause you to eat less total calories and fat during your main meal. Or, in case you don't have a chance to eat prior to your meal, order a broth-based soup or small side salad as a starter. Both contain about 150 calories, will fill you up, and lead you to eat less of your main meal.

Decide what to order ahead of time

Before you leave for a restaurant, check the online menu and decide on a few options that you can order and still work toward your target calorie deficit. Many locations now offer their nutritional facts online, but if your eatery doesn't, some safe bets are chicken, fish or lean steak with vegetables. Look out for creamy sauces and sugary marinades and glazes. If you decide ahead of time what you're going to order, you won't be easily swayed into sharing an appetizer or high-calorie entrée once you're surrounded by friends.

Did You Know?

Beware of your neighborhood chophouse! Most steak restaurants not only cook their steaks in butter, but they pour another 1/2 cup of butter over the meat at the last minute to give it that tableside sizzle. The next time you dine out, ask for your steak prepared without butter, and choose a lean cut of meat that is less than 6 ounces. Typically, anything labeled "loin" or "round" is lean. The seven leanest cuts of beef are eye round, top round, round tip, top sirloin, bottom round, top loin, and tenderloin.

Say bye-bye to the bread basket

A fast place to eliminate 100 calories or more is to stay away from the bread basket when dining out. Although you might be able to resist the rolls through willpower alone, asking the waiter to remove the bread basket from the table is more foolproof. If you were trying to quit drinking, you'd stay away from bars, right? The same goes for losing weight. Carbohydrate addiction is a real problem for many struggling dieters, because eating carbs spikes insulin and lowers blood sugar, creating the desire for even more carbs. Don't put temptation in front of you! Have the bread basket removed or, if the people you are dining with want to keep the bread basket, ask that it be moved to the far end of the table, out of your immediate reach.

Beware of "healthy" restaurant menus

Meeting friends or coworkers at Chili's, Olive Garden or Cheesecake Factory seems like a good idea — large menus with something for everyone — but they're precarious spots for someone trying to cut calories. In an attempt to appeal to people watching their calories, many restaurants have started offering "healthy" menus — Applebee's has a 550-calorie-or-less menu, Cheesecake Factory's Weight Management selections all have 600 calories or less, and Macaroni Grill recently underwent a complete menu revamp that offers healthier choices. However, a 600-calorie lunch isn't the best fit for a low-calorie plan like *Lose Up To 10 Pounds in 2 Weeks*. You want to aim for around 400 calories per main meal. Plus, these menus only really account for calories, so many of the items are super-high in fat, sugar and carbs. For example, the "Weight Management Asian Chicken Salad" from Cheesecake Factory contains 574 calories, 39 grams of fat, 68 grams of carbs, and 20 grams of sugar! You're better off sticking to meals with the fewest number of ingredients possible: grilled salmon (watch for any glazes and ask for it without them), brown rice, and steamed veggies, for instance.

Before you leave for a restaurant, check the online menu and decide on a few options that you can order and still work toward your target calorie deficit. Don't wait until you arrive, when your eyes may be bigger than your stomach.

Don't worry about what others think of what you order

When dining out, many people are so worried about what others are thinking that they order only a small side salad or whatever everyone at the table orders, only to overeat or binge on junk food later when they're alone. When they finally get to eat in the privacy of their own homes, they feel relieved and comforted by the food.

Anxiety while dining out is most prevalent in women, who often worry about being judged for eating or not appearing "ladylike" to others. "When I eat in a group, I am convinced that everyone is thinking, 'Why is she eating so much? She doesn't need to eat that,'" said one woman who admits to this behavior. But you cannot let food control you! While it is important to exert self-control when you are eating in a group, don't let others' opinions or what they are eating affect you. Stick to your diet plan, don't give in to food peer pressure, and enjoy your meal. Your company won't be assessing what or how much you ate or didn't eat — they will appreciate that you have a healthy relationship with food.

Trim Up to 500 Calories!

Pass: 22 oz. fruit smoothie, or

Swap: Veggie lasagna for meat lasagna

Don't give in to eating peer pressure

You may feel like the relaxed, social atmosphere of going out to eat with friends makes it difficult to refuse a dessert or drink. You're afraid your friends will think you're not fun if you turn down food or alcohol. It's very true that social settings create peer pressure, even among friends. People who feel the need to eat to please others or fit in will always eat more in social situations. Instead, save hundreds of calories by saying a firm "No thanks" when your dinner companions suggest splitting an appetizer or dessert. Alcohol and coffee drinks also rack up major calories, so order hot tea if everyone is having after-dinner drinks. If someone questions you, just say you don't feel like drinking alcohol and leave it at that. Remind yourself that no one will remember who ate or didn't eat what an hour after the meal, so stick to your calorie budget for that meal and never feel pressured to overindulge.

Get out of the buffet line

Buffets are tempting because of the value, the wide selection of food, and the option to go for seconds. It can be extremely difficult to practice self-control while eating a single dish, let alone resist the wide array of food, drinks, and desserts presented at buffets! The standard buffet has over 100 different options. The uncontrolled variety at buffets and the mentality that you can eat as much as you want can derail the most disciplined eater. Avoid buffet restaurants, and if the place you're dining out offers a buffet special to accompany their menu, always opt to order from the menu.

People who feel the need to eat to please others or fit in will always eat more in social situations. Instead, save hundreds of calories by saying a firm "No thanks" when your dinner companions suggest splitting an appetizer or dessert.

Veggies on the side can't be buttered or fried

Just because you chose the side of vegetables over the side of French fries, don't pat yourself on the back quite yet. A side of vegetables is only the low-calorie option if you insist on having them prepared the right way. Unfortunately, the easiest way for restaurants to cook typical side-dish veggies like zucchini, carrots, and broccoli to taste great is to sauté them in butter and salt. It's a bad sign when vegetables come served on a small side plate — they're probably soaking in butter. The extra plate keeps the melted butter-runoff contained and separate from your main meal. Veggies bathed in butter or battered and fried mean hundreds of extra calories and tons of saturated fat.

To keep them healthy and delicious, ask for your veggies steamed, sautéed in a touch of olive oil, or roasted. Don't feel guilty about sending them back if they come prepared in an unhealthy way! And when you cook them at home, try a splash of lemon juice, a drizzle of balsamic vinegar or a twist of black pepper before oven-baking vegetables like cauliflower or sweet potatoes.

Enjoy the company of friends while eating healthy by hosting a dinner party where you cook a majority of the dishes and provide the beverages. Organizing a group meal in your home means consuming hundreds of calories less than if you were heading out to a restaurant.

Resist the sales pitch

Servers are trained to describe their dishes in very appealing terms. Plus, many restaurants offer employees bonuses if they sell non-entrée items such as dessert, appetizers, and specialty drinks. For example, instead of asking, "What would you like to drink?" they may say, "We have a frozen strawberry margarita that would be perfect with some chips and guacamole." Or, a server may bring by a dessert tray or drop off a dessert menu with tempting photos without even being asked. Restaurants know hunger is very visual, so seeing a slice of cake often translates into ordering it. Don't fall into this trap that ends up adding hundreds of extra calories to your day. Politely tell your sever that you are not interested in looking at the dessert menu and not to bring the dessert tray by. Stick to your game plan and order only the items that stay within your calorie budget.

Host your own dinner party

Enjoy the company of friends while eating healthy by hosting a dinner party where you cook a majority of the dishes and provide the beverages. Cooking at home means eating smaller portions and up to 50 percent fewer calories than you would at a restaurant, and you can control what goes into each dish. This is a big benefit when you consider that many restaurant meals are prepared with unhealthy oils, butter, and creamy sauces. Serve courses that include fruits, vegetables, lean meats and whole grains, such as recipes taken from Mediterranean cuisine. Serve natural sparkling water, like Perrier, with several choices of garnish to avoid the empty calories of alcohol. Guests can feel free to bring wine or beer, but you'll have an option for sticking to your weight-loss program. Organizing a group meal in your home means consuming hundreds of calories less than if you were heading out to a restaurant and you can still spend an evening socializing with friends.

"Success means having the courage, the determination, and the will to become the person you believe you were meant to be."

~ George A. Sheehan

Chapter 10

Adopting Habits of Slim People

Do you have a friend who always passes on dessert, while you count down the minutes to treating yourself to a cookie or ice cream at the end of the day? What about someone in your family who loses 10 pounds without even trying, while you struggle with all your might just to lose a couple of pounds? It seems that all of us know at least one person who has an easy time losing weight, or even more infuriating, someone who is so naturally thin that he or she has never even had to think about it at all! Part of this person's easy relationship with their weight can be attributed to genes; indeed, some of us simply inherit high metabolic rates or extremely lean and muscular body types, which offer natural weight-loss advantages.

Yet naturally slender people also tend to have different lifestyles than do those who need to actively try to lose weight. They are less likely to use food as an emotional crutch or to resort to eating when bored, nervous, or tired. They are also more likely to be naturally drawn to physical activities that keep their metabolisms high and their muscles working. Most important,

Stay Motivated!
"Make the most of yourself, for that is
all there is of you."
~ Ralph Waldo Emerson

they tend to think differently about hunger, and thus make different choices when considering what foods to eat, when to eat them, and how much of them to eat.

What works for naturally thin people can also work for you as you continue to change your habits and lifestyle. Genetics do play a role; however, adopting the habits of thin, healthy individuals can help you to lose 10 pounds better and faster than you thought possible. Take the negative connotations away from the word "diet" and think of this program, instead, as mimicking the powerful and proven habits of slim, healthy people.

Never fall into the fad-diet trap, however. Celebrity or Hollywood diets, system cleanses, and outlandish weight-loss claims sound too good to be true — because they are. Fad diets aren't a lifestyle, they're a quick fix, and even then, many won't give you any results. And the ones that do aren't healthy. It isn't smart or wise to eat nothing but grapefruit or cereal for two meals of the day. You won't be getting the energy and nutrients you need, you'll feel sluggish, and you'll put the weight right back on when you're done with the fad diet. When you read health magazines, pay little attention to ads for fad diets or articles on celebrity weight loss and look for the "real reader success stories." These men and women have generally lost weight in a healthy way and have continued to keep it off. These are the diets and workout tips to model yourself after. These formerly overweight individuals have learned just what you will in this chapter: how to eat, exercise, and think like a thin person.

Choose being satisfied over being stuffed

Most people who are able to maintain their weight finish eating when they feel neither hungry nor full. Those who are overweight tend to continue eating past the point of comfort. The next time you eat, periodically stop and put down your utensils. Notice how your stomach feels. Can you stop eating now and feel satisfied? Find out if it is true hunger or habit that is driving you to finish your meal. If you are used to eating past the point of comfort, gradually cut back on portions and eat more slowly until you get used to stopping at a comfortable level.

Don't view hunger as good or bad

Hunger is just your body's natural signal to fuel itself. People tend to read into their hunger more than they need to. Thin people look at hunger as a simple signal from their bodies that they need food for energy. People who overeat and are overweight tend to either look forward to every meal, snack, and treat or completely dread every time they eat, fretting over every calorie. They consistently overeat or eat even when they don't have any physical signals to do so. Thin people recognize their hunger and understand where these sensations are coming from. If you find yourself eating for no reason, try skipping a snack. You may realize that you didn't even need it.

> People who overeat tend to either look forward to every meal, snack, and treat or completely dread every time they eat, fretting over every calorie. They eat even when they don't have any physical signals to do so. Thin people look at food as fuel and recognize their hunger and understand where these sensations are coming from.

Eat more fruit

A study based on the nutritional habits of slim people showed that they have an additional serving of fruit, consume more fiber, and have less fat per day than people who are overweight. The additional serving of fruit may account for the difference in weight since fruit is naturally low-fat and high in fiber. Its bulk and sweetness may satisfy lean people with a lot less calories than the cookies and pastries consumed by heavier individuals. Try to include at least 3 to 5 servings of fruit each day. Keep easy-to-eat fruits that are low on the glycemic index — meaning they cause the smallest changes to blood sugar and insulin levels — in visible places in your kitchen and office so they are handy for when you need a snack. Grapefruit, apples, cherries and pears are great choices.

Exercise an important muscle — your self control

One of the most significant behavioral indicators of weight is the amount of self-control a person has. Studies show that people who have fine-tuned their self-restraint have the lowest BMI. On the flip side, a low level of restraint has been linked to weight gain of up to 30 pounds. Your willpower is just like a muscle in that it gets stronger the more you use it! Learn to control your appetite. Plan ahead for situations where you have traditionally lacked self-control, such as celebrations and social events. Decide in advance what you will and will not eat. Pass on alcohol since it lowers inhibitions. You can't always control what is served; your willpower is sometimes all you've got.

Don't tempt yourself!

You're tying to burn or cut a significant number of calories a day to lose up to 10 pound, thus, now is not the time to be testing your willpower. Don't tempt yourself by strolling through the frozen pizza section or chip and soda aisles at the grocery store. You know what your triggers are by now, be it baked goods or the grab-and-go candy bars at the supermarket checkout. Don't spend *any* time in those aisles. If you must be in the area, don't linger, and put your "bad-food blinders" on. Get what you need and move on. And don't push the limits by thinking you'll have just a few bites of birthday cake or just one or two cookies from a package. Eating the fatty, sugary foods you love sends pleasure signals to your brain and stopping at just a bite or two will be nearly impossible. Why take the risk?

Keep easy-to-eat fruits that are low on the glycemic index — meaning they cause the smallest changes to blood sugar and insulin levels — in visible places in your kitchen and office so they are handy for when you need a snack. Grapefruit, apples, cherries and pears are great choices.

Get moving!

Studies indicate that slim people move around several hours a week more than those who are overweight. This extra activity can account for an additional weight loss of 2 to 3 pounds! How much do you move around during the day? If you have a desk job, you might spend a large portion of your day sitting — although you don't have to. Get up and move around as much as you can. Walk around while talking on the phone; take the stairs up and down a few times; walk to the other side of the office to talk to a coworker in person, rather than sending an email. Your day should involve taking 10,000 steps a day. This type of activity is extremely valuable to your body's "non-exercise activity thermogenesis," or NEAT, which is the calorie burning process that happens naturally from everyday movements such as standing up, fidgeting, turning, bending and walking. A physically active person burns approximately 30 percent of their calories through daily "non-intentional exercise," versus 15 percent for sedentary people. Try to incorporate other physical activities into your day, such as vacuuming, shopping, or playing with your kids or dog.

Ask yourself, is it worth it?

Thin people evaluate what they eat based on how hard they will have to exercise to burn off the extra calories. If you are considering splurging on a piece of cheesecake, for instance, consider that you'll need to run for 45 minutes to get back to where your calorie count was prior to eating it. That's just to break even! And when you're looking to create a calorie deficit each day, you'll be way behind if you have that dessert. Ask yourself, do you want to negate a good, sweaty gym session with a few bites of food? Think thin and say no to any snack, drink, or treat that will mean extra hours of exercise (or depriving yourself of nutritious food) to compensate. In the end, you'll realize it just isn't worth it.

Trim Up to 200 Calories!
Pass: Side of potato or macaroni salad, or
Swap: Chicken broth instead of butter for cooking veggies

Get some ZZZZZs

Statistically, people who have less body fat get about 2 more hours of sleep a week versus those who are overweight. Researchers suggest that increased body weight from lack of sleep is linked to our hormones. Sleep deprivation decreases the amounts of leptin in our system, the hormone that suppresses hunger, and increases the levels of ghrelin, an appetite-boosting hormone. Cravings for salty and sugary foods increase and motivation to stay away from high-calorie foods decreases. Thin people tend to get between 7 and 9 hours of sleep a night. Give yourself the best shot at a great day of healthy eating by going to bed 15 to 30 minutes earlier than your typical bedtime. If you have trouble settling into bed, a warm bath or mug of non-caffeinated tea can help (warm liquids are soothing). Also, be sure to put away your electronics 30 minutes before you get into bed. Checking emails, browsing the Internet, and text messaging can make it hard to fall asleep.

> A physically active person burns approximately 30 percent of their calories through daily "non-intentional exercise," versus 15 percent for sedentary people.

Don't forget about your diet on the weekends

People who maintain their weight follow their diet game plan 7 days of the week. Saturdays and Sundays aren't free rein to forget about smart eating and overindulge. To lose significant weight each week, you need to resist lazy-weekend temptations: beer-soaked sporting events, late-night pizza binges, and calorie-packed pancake brunches. Too often you'll hear dieters call one day of the week their "cheat day," but consider that eating an extra 500 calories on Saturday may mean having to create a 2,000-calorie deficit on another day. It's just not smart or healthy. Maintaining similar eating patterns for all days of the week will help you establish healthy choices as long-term habits. Don't forget to plan your meals for the entire week ahead of time. This will keep you from wavering from your eating plan on the weekends.

Always ask for dressing on the side

As a rule of thumb: Don't ever trust restaurant salad dressings! Smart eaters know that even the light-sounding dressings on restaurant menus, such as raspberry vinaigrette or Asian sesame vinaigrette, for instance, are full of sugar. And restaurants are infamous for pouring on far too much dressing. A weight-loss tip: Dip your fork into the dressing cup several times and spread it over the salad. You'll get the flavor of the dressing without soaking your salad and adding tons of calories. And, if you don't douse your salad with a full cup of dressing, you can take part of it home to eat that night or the next day.

Tune out advertising

Thin people learn to tune out food advertisements and stick with their eating plans, no matter what special combo meal is now available. Be aware of how food ads affect you, and you'll be one step closer to thinking thin and putting an end to mindless snacking.

Online, on TV, or simply driving down the road, you are exposed to dozens of advertisements for food each day. An interesting study from the Rudd Center for Food Policy and Obesity at Yale showed that people are profoundly affected by food advertising and that these effects occur regardless of people's initial hunger. The study measured the amount of snack foods consumed during and after advertising exposure and found that both children and adults consumed significantly more of both healthy and unhealthy snack foods following exposure to snack food advertising. Additionally, food advertising increased consumption of all available foods, even foods that were not presented in the advertisements, contradicting food industry claims that advertising affects only brand preferences and not overall nutrition. Jennifer Harris, one of the authors of the study, concluded,

"Food advertising triggers automatic eating, regardless of hunger, and is a significant contributor to the obesity epidemic."

Stay alert when food advertisements pop up around you. Thin people learn to tune them out and stick with their eating plans, no matter what special combo meal is now available at a neighborhood restaurant. Observe correlations between snacking and emotional hunger and advertisements. Be aware of how food ads affect you, and you'll be one step closer to thinking thin and putting an end to mindless snacking.

Statistically, people who have less body fat get about 2 more hours of sleep a week versus those who are overweight.

Practice positive visualization

Ask yourself, "What is stopping me from losing weight?" Do you believe you're doomed to fail? Do you start your diet imagining all the foods you'll miss or how hungry you'll surely be? Thin, healthy, fit people look at eating well and exercising as a lifestyle, not a punishment or a constant battle. Practice being positive about your new program from the get-go. Disassociate your eating plan with restriction and deprivation. Instead, view it as enjoying the right foods in the right amounts. Now, visualize your happier, healthier, thinner self after losing 10 pounds. Picture yourself in a swimsuit, lying in the warm sun on the beach, feeling confident. Visualize yourself cooking and enjoying a healthy dinner with friends or family. Imagine yourself walking into a party full of people and how they'll all notice your new body, confidence and happiness. You can literally feel how proud you will be. Positive visualization reinforces the reasons you're losing weight and keeps your eye on the prize.

“ Self-image sets the boundaries of individual accomplishment. ”

~ Maxwell Maltz

Chapter 11

Secrets to Lose Weight At-A-Glance

This book is full of tips and secrets for slimming down, tightening up, and looking and feeling better every day. The following section contains 100 diet secrets that you can refer to at-a-glance whenever you need motivation or a reminder of the most effective principles for eating right and losing weight.

This is a great section to look back on after the 2 weeks, as well, since it gives you dozens of tips, tricks and important pieces of advice on eating to lose weight, right at your fingertips. "Diet" doesn't have to be a dirty word; you just have to know the secrets of what to eat, how much, and how often.

Happy healthy eating!

SECRETS TO LOSE WEIGHT AT-A-GLANCE

1. **Identify your ideal weight.** Having a specific goal in mind will keep your eye on the prize!

2. **Expect to lose weight over time.** Amazing results won't happen overnight, but you'll see real changes in your body and energy levels with the secrets in this book after just a few days.

3. **Figure out the factors that determine your weight.** Place effort into changing what you can control, such as the food you eat and how much you exercise. Don't waste time and energy trying to change aspects of your appearance that are determined by age or body type.

4. **Learn to eyeball portion sizes.** Associate proper portions for foods you like to eat with the size of common objects so you eat just the right amount.

5. **Know how your age affects the rate at which you lose weight.** It's never too late to create healthy eating habits. Maintain a balanced body composition and learn how to eat smart to ward off health risks.

6. **Modify your diet and exercise plan as you lose weight.** The more weight you lose, the fewer calories you will burn during exercise, so adjust your diet to include foods that fill you up longer with fewer calories.

7. **Focus on both short-term and long-term goals.** Short-term goals will allow you to witness the more immediate results of your hard work. Breaking down your program into smaller, more focused intervals will make goals seem within your reach.

8. **Figure out the serving sizes for your favorite foods.** The key to weight loss is every food in moderation. If you love pasta, for instance, it's important to know the proper serving size so you know exactly how many calories you're eating.

9. **Calculate your daily calorie allowance.** Multiply your Basal Metabolic Rate (BMR) by the number that corresponds to your activity level to get your calorie allowance.
   1.200 = sedentary
   1.375 = lightly active, 1-3 days/week
   1.550 = moderately active, 3-5 days/week
   1.725 = very active, 6-7 days a week
   1.900 = extra active, sport/physical job

10. **Create a calorie deficit.** The only way to lose weight is the create a daily calorie deficit, meaning that you expend more calories through diet and exercise than you take in. A minimum of a 500-calorie deficit per day is required to lose 1 pound per week.

11. **Find out how many calories are in your favorite foods.** Studies show that people drastically underestimate the number of calories in the foods they eat. Look at nutrition labels, buy a calorie counting book, and search online restaurant menus to know what's in the foods you're ordering and making.

12. **Incorporate foods from each of the six main food groups into your diet plan.** A balanced diet means that you'll be getting the right nutrients to stay active and energized. Be sure you're meeting the USDA standards for each of the six food groups.

13. **Understand the type of diets available.** Create a diet plan that is tailored to your lifestyle and personal preferences. Avoid fad and celebrity diets that restrict food to dangerous levels or eliminate whole food groups.

14. **Don't totally deprive yourself of your favorite foods.** Going cold turkey with the foods you love will lead you to feel deprived and cause binges. Find healthy substitutions or allow yourself the foods you crave in small amounts.

15. **Change the way you look at diets.** Disassociate dieting with restriction and deprivation. Look at dieting as eating the right foods in the right amounts.

16. **Be committed to losing weight.** It's too easy to give up once your diet plan gets tough. Commit yourself to the full 2 weeks and watch how it becomes easier each day.

17. **Make losing weight a priority.** Grocery shopping, cooking at home, and exercising all take time, so make these a priority, just as you would a meeting or appointment. Make time to lose weight!

18. **Buy 100-calorie snack packs.** Snack the right way with 100-calorie packs of nuts, crackers, carrots, chips, and more. Or, make your own!

19. **Create good habits to reach your goal.** You will be amazed at how many eating choices are simply what you're used to doing, instead of what you know is smart. Concentrate on a few new behaviors at the beginning of each week.

20. **Seek expert advice.** Your doctor will be able to help if you have specific dietary needs, such as diabetes or food allergies, or if you are a vegetarian. Consult a dietetics professional on how you can safely lose weight and develop an appropriate eating plan.

21. **Talk to a professional if you have a past history of disordered eating.** If you have had an eating disorder, a professional should coach you through the best way to eat better without diving back into disordered habits.

22. **Keep tempting foods out of sight and out of mind.** If you don't have the high-calorie foods you crave around your house or in your desk at work, then you won't be tempted to eat them when hunger strikes.

23. **Follow basic nutritional guidelines.** Eat at least 60 grams of protein to build and repair body tissue. Include a minimum of 100 grams of carbohydrates daily to avoid feeling fatigued. Make sure you get 20 to 30 grams of fiber to aid in digestion.

24. **Strive for consistency with your weight-loss program.** Consistent behaviors will enable you to lose weight. Don't overeat one day and overcompensate the next by starving yourself.

25. **Combine calorie reduction and increased activity to lose weight.** You can't lose 10 pounds and keep it off with diet alone! Diet and fitness are a powerful fat-fighting combination.

26. **Take a walk to beat hunger.** You may be eating out of boredom. When cravings strike, go for a short 15-minute walk to fend off hunger.

27. **Make sure your diet plan includes enough calories.**
If you don't get enough calories, you will feel lethargic, without enough energy to participate in your fitness plan. The American College of Sports Medicine (ACSM) recommends that calorie levels don't drop below 1,200 calories per day for women or 1,800 calories for men.

28. **Don't rely on a weight-loss plan that eliminates carbohydrates.** Your body needs complex carbs because they are the energy source for the brain and red blood cells. For focus, energy and stamina for exercise and your day, eat unrefined carbs.

29. **Find weight-loss solutions that do not involve crash dieting.** Losing weight on a crash diet is often the result of decreased muscle mass and water loss. When normal eating patterns are resumed, people gain the weight back. Strive for a healthier diet that keeps you full longer, plus daily exercise.

30. **Be wary of diet plans that sound too good to be true.**
Learn how to distinguish a fad diet from a sensible one. Fad diets often exclude foods necessary for good health and do not instruct the dieter to build healthy eating habits.

31. **Make small changes to see big results.** Consider this: Saving just 100 calories every day would mean losing 10 pounds a year. Go for a brisk walk, cut out soda and cut back on cheese and mayo at lunch. Little changes go a long way.

32. **Stay hydrated.** People often think they are hungry when they are actually thirsty. Drink at least 8 or 9 full glasses of water throughout the day to stave off hunger pangs.

33. **Splurge wisely.** Diets become overwhelming if you don't allow for some flexibility. Give yourself a planned break every once in a while. Figure out what you can enjoy without undermining your weight loss.

34. **Give yourself enough time to burn off your evening meal.** Eat at least 3 hours before bedtime. Take a brisk walk after dinner, or do some chores, light exercising, or stretching to help burn off your evening meal.

35. **Limit the number of carbohydrates you eat at night.** If you want to lose weight, consider eating fewer carbohydrates, such as white bread, chips, and cookies, before you go to bed. You are more likely to store fat when eating carb-rich foods at night.

36. **Do not buy anything mega-, super-, or king sized.** Never succumb to the fast-food trap of meals that come with super-sized upgrades. You'll save hundreds of calories by saying, "No thanks" when prompted at the drive-thru window.

37. **Eat low-density, high water-content foods to fill you up without weight gain**. High-fiber foods, such as non-starchy vegetables, high water-content fruits, fat-free milk, fish, and lean proteins have low calorie content and high water content, meaning you can fill up on them without added calories.

38. **Let healthy eating become a way of life.** You probably don't crave broccoli and lettuce; no one does. But once you make it a habit to eat healthy, fresh foods every day, you will want to continue clean eating. Eating a sugary candy bar won't even sound appetizing.

39. **Beware of trans fats.** Consumption of trans fats promotes heart disease, cancer, diabetes, immune dysfunction, and reproductive problems. Avoid candy, chips, packaged snacks, pastries, donuts, cookies, and fried foods.

40. **Know the difference between psychological and physical hunger.** The body gives cues and clues to physical hunger, whereas psychological hunger is triggered by emotions. Learn the difference to eat only when hungry.

41. **Eat at least 5 servings of fruits and vegetables per day.** Fruits and vegetables have high fiber and water content, which means they fill you up and keep you full longer.

42. **Serve your food hot.** Foods served hot can be more satiating, so you are likely to eat less. And, when food is hot, you have to take time to eat it.

43. **Shift in your seat.** Fidgeting can burn up to 350 calories a day. Swing or bounce your legs, and tap your feet or fingers. Alternate between flexing and relaxing your muscles or shift your weight from side to side.

44. **Read the label.** People don't pay enough attention to nutritional labels when choosing foods. Check out the serving size, servings per container, calories, saturated fat, calories from fat, and sodium for every product you eat.

45. **Focus on the positive.** Acknowledge your good qualities and tell yourself that you are making yourself even better by losing weight. This will keep you motivated on the tough days.

46. **Get enough rest.** People who don't get enough sleep tend to be overweight and crave caloric and fatty foods. Proper sleep regulates the hormones that tell your body you are hungry or full, so get 7 to 9 hours a night.

47. **Eat low density, high volume foods.** Eat the same amount of food you usually do, but fill up on low-calorie, high volume foods, such as fruits, vegetables, soups, stews, cooked grains, lean meats, fish, and lean poultry.

48. **Ditch soda.** If you are drinking a soda with each meal, this can amount to 300 or more extra calories a day. Simply drinking water instead of these sodas amounts to about 1 pound of weight loss per week.

49. **Consider your resolution to lose weight as a benefit to yourself, not a test of your willpower.** Constantly pressuring yourself to be perfect can lead you to feel overwhelmed. Instead of viewing diets as a constant source of stress, consider losing weight as something good that you are doing for yourself.

50. **Know that organic isn't healthier by nature.** Organic food is simply grown and produced without harsh chemicals, but the calories in organic products are no different than conventional ones. Don't fall into that diet trap. An organic pie is still made with butter and oil.

51. **Limit processed foods.** Processed foods are refined carbohydrates devoid of essential vitamins and minerals and often high in calories. These foods are quickly digested and leave us feeling hungry shortly after eating them.

52. **Decrease stress.** Hormones produced under stress, such as cortisol and epinephrine, can lead to fat storage around the abdomen. Adopt some relaxation techniques such as yoga or deep breathing to reduce your stress levels and lose weight.

53. **Choose carbohydrates wisely.** Choose complex carbohydrates found in whole grains, fruits, and vegetables, which provide a low release of energy so your body has a greater chance to burn off calories before they get stored as fat.

54. **Don't eat more of low-fat items.** Studies have shown that people tend to overeat when they know that an item is low-fat or fat-free. Don't fall into this trip. Set aside a pre-portioned amount of every snack you eat.

55. **Drink 5 cups of green tea daily.** Antioxidant-packed green tea helps you drop pounds by increasing fat oxidation and thermogenesis, the process where your body temperature increases as a result of burning fat. Green tea can also prevent the storage of excess sugar and fat in the body.

56. **Check food label claims.** Products that are labeled as "low-fat" or "reduced" often include other high-calorie ingredients. Check the label to make sure the product does not contain extra sugar or fat.

57. **Increase your calorie-burning potential by eating small meals throughout the day.** You burn calories with every meal as your body digests food. Keep your metabolism doing its job by spreading out large meals into smaller ones consumed throughout the day.

58. **Use smaller plates and bowls.** Filling up a smaller plate or bowl gives the impression you're eating more when you're actually eating less. Eating with small utensils also forces you to eat more slowly.

59. **Pour drinks into taller, thinner glasses.** If you pour drinks into short, wide glasses, chances are you serve yourself up to 30 percent more than you think. Switch to taller, narrow glasses to keep from drinking extra calories.

60. **Define your incentive to lose weight.** Give yourself an incentive to eat healthy, even when you're tempted to snack and overeat. Choose an event that you would like to lose weight for, such as your birthday, a vacation, or a social event.

61. **Eat spicy foods.** Spicy foods, primarily red pepper, cayenne, and chili pepper, may help raise your metabolism by around 8 percent for up to 2 to 3 hours after eating.

62. **Eat at regular intervals.** Eating at regular intervals aids in controlling hunger and prevents overeating later in the day when you are less likely to have time to burn off extra calories.

63. **Leave extras off salads and sandwiches.** Pass on cheese, mayo, bacon, and croutons when ordering salads and sandwiches. Chances are, you won't even miss them, and you'll save hundreds of calories.

64. **Balance your energy levels.** Eat first thing in the morning and before you exercise to prevent your body from breaking down muscle tissue for energy.

65. **Don't be a slave to the scale.** Day to day changes in your weight can be misleading or discouraging. Weigh yourself first thing in the morning, without clothes, and recognize that water retention and muscle gain can cause weight gain.

66. **Tell your friends and family.** Let the people in your life know that you have decided to lose weight. Tell them what kinds of foods you can eat and the foods you want to avoid. Tell them that you need to eat less and not to put pressure on you to eat more.

67. **Join a weight-loss support group.** Look for local or online communities where you can share your story, get weight-loss tips, and ask for advice. These groups are educational, give you a sense of accountability, and provide a sense of community.

68. **Make a shopping list and stick to it.** Focus on only the items you need to lose weight and stick with the items you have pre-selected as part of your diet program.

69. **Resist last-minute temptations when you check out.** Check-out aisles are laden with foods that are high in fat, calories, sugar, and salt. Plan ahead and remind yourself to have willpower.

70. **Celebrate successes.** Reward yourself for sticking to your diet plan throughout your weight-loss journey. Get a massage or manicure, buy a new book, or see a movie. Choose a reward that's not food-related.

71. **Cook and eat meals at home.** Prepare your own meals as often as you can. You can control exactly what goes into each meal if you make it yourself.

72. **Be prepared for roadblocks.** You may encounter obstacles, such as a party or dinner out that you think may lead to overeating. Plan ahead for such occasions so you're not caught off-guard by food.

73. **Enjoy snacks with protein and carbs for all-day energy.** Snacks like hummus and veggies or all-natural peanut butter and whole grain crackers will give you energy to get through your day better than a bag of chips or fruit or vegetables alone.

74. **Realize that the last 10 pounds can be the most challenging to lose.** Shedding the last 10 pounds requires shaking up your current lifestyle. Sticking to this 14-day plan isn't easy, but the results will be worth it.

75. **Make smart snack swaps.** Instead of a bag of Skittles, for instance, satisfy your sweet and sour tastebuds with a half of a grapefruit lightly sprinkled with brown sugar.

76. **Keep healthy staples in the fridge.** Have the following basic items available at all times: chicken and fish; fruits and vegetables that can be eaten easily, such as baby carrots, celery sticks, apples, strawberries, and grapes; bagged lettuce for salads; low-fat milk and yogurt; eggs or an egg substitute; and whole grain breads and high-fiber, low-sugar cereal.

77. **Keep a list of healthy foods, snacks, and meals you enjoy.** Many people feel like they have nothing to eat when they are losing weight. Write down a list to make shopping easy. Use this book's reusable grocery list to take the guesswork out of choosing healthy products and ingredients.

78. **Eat breakfast.** Skipping breakfast will actually train your body to store fat when it senses you are not getting enough food. Jumpstart your metabolism and energy levels with "the most important meal of the day."

79. **Eat natural or whole foods.** Create a diet that focuses on whole foods such as fruit, vegetables, whole grains, and legumes. Because they are high in complex carbohydrates and fiber, they are digested slowly.

80. **Add lean protein to your diet.** Proteins help build muscles and can increase your metabolic rate, because the energy it takes to digest and absorb protein accounts for approximately 25 percent of the total calories protein contains.

81. **Burn more calories than you eat with nutrient, fiber-dense foods like fruits and vegetables.** The high fiber content in fruits and veggies requires more energy to digest than the amount of calories in the foods themselves, so add as many of these foods to your diet as possible.

82. **Shop for groceries when you are not hungry.** Stop by the grocery store after a large meal when you won't be as likely to stray from your shopping list. Or, drink a large glass of water beforehand.

83. **Create a dietary itinerary to lose weight while traveling.** Look up healthy restaurants in the area you're visiting. Also, ask for the minibar in your room to be emptied. Shop for a few foods to keep in your room to avoid temptation to order room service.

84. **Don't view hunger as good or bad.** Hunger is just your body's natural signal to fuel itself. Try to look at hunger as a simple signal from your body that you need food for energy.

85. **Keep some meal replacement options in your car and at work.** Look for bars or shakes that contain no more than 5 to 7 grams of fat, at least 3 to 5 grams of fiber, around 15 grams of protein, and 35 percent of your daily allowance of vitamins and minerals.

86. **Prepare your own meals in advance.** Prepare meals and snacks ahead of time to make sure that a healthy option is always available. For example, when cooking fish or chicken for dinner, make a few extra pieces and use them in salads or tacos the next day.

87. **Identify your hunger.** Figure out if you are experiencing true physical hunger, low blood sugar hunger, cravings, comfort eating, or social hunger. Find reasonable ways to deal with each situation.

88. **Navigate stores with efficiency.** Navigate the periphery of the store where fresh meat, fish, and produce are stocked. Avoid the aisles with the most tempting foods, such as chips, cookies, candy, and pastries.

89. **Take note of the relationships between food and mood.** When you fill out your diet journal, look for relationships between what and when you eat and how you feel. This will give you clues to where you can cut back or change what you're eating.

90. **Don't rule out foods because of the time of day.** You'll have more healthy options if you break the habit of eating certain foods only at specific times of day. A hard-boiled egg with a bowl of oatmeal and fruit can be a great lunch or dinner.

91. **Stock your freezer with healthy frozen entrees.** Healthy frozen meals contain a good ratio of carbs, protein, and fats in each meal. Select entrees that range from 200 to 400 calories with less than 10 grams of fat.

92. **Plan each week ahead of time.** Figure out what your schedule looks like for the following week and stock up on healthy options. Decide what you want to eat and make sure you purchase ingredients to prepare meals ahead of time.

93. **Plan a sweet but healthy treat.** Include a sweet treat into your weight-loss plan so you don't feel deprived, but try to keep these foods between 200 and 250 calories, such as a few Peppermint Patties or Jolly Ranchers.

94. **Find ways to stick to your diet when you are stuck on an airplane.** Have portable, healthy snacks on hand when you are caught with delays or are faced with the in-flight meal. Pack nuts, crackers, or a piece of fruit.

95. **Know what foods trigger your appetite.** Common trigger foods usually combine sugar and fat, or fat and salt. With trigger foods, a single bite can result in a binge, so avoid these foods all together. Don't allow yourself even one bite.

96. **Find ways to control your hunger.** Keep your appetite stable by eating smaller meals more often and choosing low-calorie, nutrient-dense foods, such as apples, sweet potatoes, salads, and grilled chicken.

97. **Don't eat if you are not hungry.** Our bodies are conditioned to expect food at specific times of the day. But instead of having a full dinner after eating a late lunch, have a small snack, such as a bowl of soup or an apple with a tablespoon of peanut butter.

98. **Realize that seeing foods you crave can make you want to eat them more.** Appetite is very visual. Don't linger over menus with large images of high-calorie meals and desserts. Don't let your gaze wander to other diners' plates when eating out.

99. **Steer clear of refined carbohydrates.** Carb addiction occurs when refined carbohydrates cause blood sugar to spike and then drop, making the body crave more carbs. Stay away from bagels, muffins, donuts and these types of foods.

100. **Brush your teeth after meals to halt hunger.** Brushing your teeth after eating can stop you from putting more food in your mouth. Also, peppermint flavor and smell has been shown to reduce hunger over a short period of time.

" Plant your garden and decorate your own soul, instead of waiting for someone to bring you flowers. **"**

~ Veronica A. Shoffstall

Chapter 12

Exercising to Lose Weight

Too many people falsely believe they can lose weight by simply eating less or eating better, without sweating one bit. However, creating a calorie deficit from your diet alone, without combining diet with exercise, is nearly impossible, if not dangerous. In addition, an extremely low-calorie diet means you'll lack the energy and stamina you need to get through your day. On the flip side, many people assume if they become moderately active they can lose weight without giving up their indulgences of ice cream, burritos and burgers. Unfortunately, neither is a healthy approach and neither will allow you to lose 10 pounds or reach your ideal weight.

Consider this: A University of Virginia study reported that to lose 1 pound of body fat you would have to do 250,000 sit-ups — or 100 sit-ups every day for 7 years. Exercise alone won't give you a flat stomach and defined abs — it's the layer of body fat covering your muscles that needs to be whittled away through eating low-fat, low-calorie foods and cardiovascular work that allows muscles to show.

Likewise, a Mayo Clinic report revealed the prevalence of "skinny overweight" people, or what is being called "normal weight obesity." As many as 30 million "thin" Americans are believed to have a body fat percentage that puts them in the overweight category and at risk for disease, despite appearing to be of a normal weight.

Healthy eating and exercise are a powerful fat- and disease-fighting combo and only with the combination of the two can you drop unwanted pounds and start feeling amazing.

Just an hour of exercise a day burns hundreds of calories, making meeting your goal very doable. In addition, you will find that exercise is energizing, builds muscle tone, curbs your appetite, and increases your metabolism.

Lose Up To 10 Pounds in 2 Weeks covers the importance of redefining your food choices, creating a game plan to address each meal and craving, and making healthy changes to your habits. This knowledge will help you eat hundreds of calories less a day and shed unwanted pounds; however, you can't lose 10 pounds, and keep it off, without exercise. You need to stay full and satisfied throughout the day; cutting calories through diet restriction alone may very well mean you're eating too little, and eating too little leaves the door dangerously open for bingeing.

However, including exercise in your weight-loss program means you can easily reach a substantial calorie deficit without starving yourself. Just an hour of exercise a day burns hundreds of calories, making meeting your goal very doable. In addition, you will find that exercise is energizing, builds muscle tone, curbs your appetite, and increases your metabolism.

So what is the best exercise regimen for you to embark on? The answer depends on your personality, interests, and individual abilities. You can do it all at one time or integrate it into two or three segments over the course of your day. Just be sure to build a plan that fits into your daily calendar and keep in mind that the common ingredient for any successful exercise program is to choose activities you will enjoy doing and that you may even look forward to each day.

Incorporate all three elements of fitness

Your fitness program should include all three essential elements for successful weight loss and maintenance: cardiovascular activities to burn calories, benefit your heart and reduce body fat; resistance or strength training for muscle tone; and a basic stretching routine to improve flexibility and prevent injury. Cardio is the most beneficial for weight loss and should be your main focus, but each element complements the others. Resistance and strength training will firm up muscles as the unwanted pounds melt away. Increased muscle mass will also burn extra calories throughout the day. Stretching and flexibility develop range of motion, increase muscle elasticity, achieve muscle balance, and protect the body from injury.

When you do cardio, you want to make sure you're moving continuously and getting your heart rate up. You should be breathing hard. The rule of thumb is, be working hard enough during cardio that you can answer questions but not carry on a conversation. Typical activities include jogging/running, elliptical training, bicycling/spinning, and cardio classes such as step aerobics, kickboxing, and aerobic dance. For strength training, aim for at least two 30-minute sessions per week that may include free weights, weight machines, resistance equipment, muscular endurance training, and toning activities such as Power yoga or Pilates. Focus on activities that exercise each of the major muscle groups or work more than one muscle group at the same time. Stretching is important before, during and after a workout. A study found that regular stretching can increase your strength by up to 19 percent when interspersed between weight-training exercises, for instance. Try doing 10 or 15 minutes of basic Ashtanga yoga poses.

Did You Know?

One of the best predictors of maintaining a fitness program over time is exercising in a social environment, like a gym or fitness class, or having a workout buddy. Think about it: The people you see each time you exercise become friends and acquaintances who expect to say hello to you, so you're less likely to skip a class or workout. Plus, you're making new friends while you slim down!

Create a realistic schedule you can stick to

Schedule your workouts at the beginning of the week, just like you are doing with your meals for the week. Be realistic! If you're not a morning person, don't schedule 6 a.m. runs. If you like to relax after work, don't pretend you're going to take a yoga class in the evenings. Take a look at your calendar and pencil in workouts for at least 5 days of the week, on days and times that are most doable. For instance, plan morning workouts for the days when you'll want to meet friends after work, or schedule a lunchtime hike for a day when you want to sleep in. Building exercise around your personal schedule and lifestyle means you're more likely to meet your goals.

Get a walking workout

Many people starting out a fitness plan turn to good old-fashioned walking.

On a nice day, consider a stroll around your neighborhood. In cold or rainy weather, go to the mall and log miles while you window shop. Walking is a cost-effective activity that simply requires a good pair of shoes. Walking may sound too good to be true, but it is an aerobic activity that burns calories. Consider the fact that for a 150-pound person, walking at 2 mph, which is approximately a 30-minute mile, burns 189 calories per hour. Walking a 20-minute mile at a 3 mph pace uses 300 calories per hour. Walking a moderate, 15-minute mile, for an average of 4 mph, burns 300 calories per hour. The faster you walk, the more calories you will burn.

If you're not sure how far a mile is in your neighborhood, you can drive your car while looking at your odometer or buy a small pedometer to count your steps. The U.S. Surgeon General has recommended walking 30 minutes daily to strive toward a weekly goal of 10,000 steps, or roughly 5 miles. Those on a weight-loss program should strive for a minimum of 12,000 to 15,000 steps, which should take about 45 minutes per day.

Look at your weekly schedule and be realistic! If you're not a morning person, don't schedule 6 a.m. runs. If you like to relax after work, don't pretend you're going to take a yoga class in the evenings.

Fend off food cravings with exercise

To increase your daily exercise and stave off cravings and hunger pangs, go for a walk the next time you feel like eating when it's not a snack or meal time. People often snack when they need a break from work or family, or when they're bored. Instead, try going for a 15-minute walk and allowing the craving to pass. Walking for 15 minutes will burn 75 calories for a 150-pound person. So, instead of eating a 150-calorie snack out of boredom, you'll have actually burned calories!

Find solutions to your exercise excuses

There are many excuses to skip exercise or to let a fitness plan fall by the wayside after a short time. But you won't be able to lose weight without exercise to complement a reduced-calorie diet. Get out a piece of paper and write down the reasons you've been avoiding exercise, joining a gym, or taking a fitness class. Some of the most common reasons people use to avoid physical activity include:

"I don't have the time."
"I'm too tired and I don't feel like it."
"I'm not very good at exercising."
"It's not convenient to get to my workout place."
"I'm afraid and embarrassed."
"It's too expensive to join a gym."

Trim Up to 500 Calories!
Pass: Tuna deli sub, or
Swap: Sparkling fruit-flavored water instead of champagne

Now write down solutions to these excuses. For example, if your number one reason for skipping exercise is "I don't have time," use half your lunch break to go for a brisk walk or take a bike ride with your family instead of seeing a movie (you'll still spend time together, get to interact, and do something good for everyone's health). The bottom line is, there is never a good excuse to be sedentary. There are great gyms and fitness facilities of all types and price ranges. If you find the traditional gym environment isn't for you, try a cycling club or dance class. If money is a concern, sign up for a hiking club — things like hiking, swimming, and rollerblading are always free. There are hundreds of ways to burn calories, so stop making excuses — make time and find something you like to do.

Take measures to avoid injury

Nothing puts a cramp in your weight loss like an injury. And if it's something serious enough, it can even mean the end of your exercise plan all together. There are several ways to avoid injury when you're embarking on a new fitness plan. Always warm up and cool down for at least 5 to 10 minutes, before and after workouts. Warm up is especially important if you're doing early morning cardio because your body will be completely cold — like giving a car a chance to warm up after it's been sitting in a garage overnight. Also, give your body time to rest in between workouts. Get in a few hard workouts but then take one day off completely each week. For strength training, take at least one day off between sessions that work the same muscle group so you give the muscle fibers time to heal and strengthen. Finally, be sure you ask a trainer the proper form and technique for exercises and machines that are new to you to avoid pulling or straining a muscle.

The best way to see your progress and maintain motivation is keeping track of the days you exercise in the 2-week journal in the back of this book. Seeing the days accumulate on your calendar will really keep you motivated for the times when the gym sounds less than tempting.

Use your fitness journal!

In order to lose up to 10 pounds in 2 weeks, you need to expend more calories per day more than you eat. Therefore, exercise must become a part of your daily and weekly routine. The best way to see your progress and maintain motivation is keeping track of the days you exercise in the 2-week journal in the back of this book. Seeing the days accumulate on your calendar will really keep you motivated for the times when the gym sounds less than tempting. Write down the activity you did, the duration of time, reps, and the intensity (or weight, if strength training). Keep track of everything you do, and don't underestimate what may seem like a smaller activity, such as walking your dog. Consider that a 150-pound person will burn 100 calories from just a 20-minute walk at a moderate pace. Every little bit counts, just like with calories, so write it down and applaud yourself for making time throughout the day to get moving.

> Consider a virtual trainer — a real person who will create a fitness plan specifically for you, based on your goals and the equipment you have available to you. You'll get online tutorials, text message reminders, and email check-ins from your trainer.

Join an online weight-loss community

Create a profile page at an online weight-loss and fitness community and you'll have instant access to a huge group of people with similar goals, questions, obstacles, and tips for success. Seeing what works for others gives you motivation, and hearing about the ups and downs of exercise and losing weight from real people provides comfort and a sense of solidarity.

Enlist a virtual trainer

Hiring a personal trainer can be a great motivator and learning experience but not everyone is ready for the time or money commitment it requires. A terrific option is a virtual trainer. A real person will create a fitness plan specifically for you, based on your goals and the equipment you have available to you. You'll get online tutorials on the proper form for exercises, worksheets for tracking progress, and accountability in the form of reminders and check-ins from your virtual trainer.

Never give up!

"Don't give up, don't ever give up," legendary college basketball coach

Jim Valvano told the crowd at the 1993 ESPY Awards, a night to celebrate the accomplishments of the greatest athletes in the world. Inspired by Valvano's fight against bone cancer, the athletes in the room also knew plenty about the resilience it takes to stay in top shape and perform under the most pressure imaginable. Valvano's words should inspire you, too!

Losing weight is a journey that takes determination and resilience, and exercise can be struggle if you haven't always been active. If you have had a busy day of work or family, it is tempting to spend an evening on the couch instead of going for a run or bike ride. One of the toughest things is getting back on an exercise schedule after you've missed a few days. But don't decide you've failed. If you skip a day of your workout, tell yourself you'll start again tomorrow. If you overindulge at a meal, be firm that you will have a longer, tougher workout the next day. If you feel like skipping the gym, tell yourself you'll do 30 minutes (odds are, you'll stay longer). Don't give up!

"Without discipline, there's no life at all."
~ Katharine Hepburn

Chapter 13

Maximizing Your Workouts

To lose up to 10 pounds in a short amount of time you need to make the most of every workout or physical activity you do. You don't want to do the same exercises or routine every day for 2 weeks. To optimize the amount of calories and body fat you burn during each workout and lose as much weight as you can, use the tips and tricks in this chapter to learn when and how to work out, how to dress for your chosen activity, and how to stay motivated on days when you're feeling sluggish or lazy.

There is a lot to learn and remember when starting an intense fitness program like this one. In this chapter, you'll learn the right amount of weight you should be lifting during strength training, how to calculate your maximum and target heart rates, find how much water you should be drinking, and determine the best time to get new shoes and which type to buy.

Use the tips, formulas, and principles of fitness in this chapter to maximize your workout results. Nothing will make you feel better or more excited to maintain your program. With 2 weeks to go to lose up to 10 pounds, you have no time to waste!

Work the "afterburn"

Do cardiovascular exercise first thing in the morning! During the night, your body becomes depleted of your primary energy source, carbohydrates. With that in short supply, your body begins to work from its secondary source, which is body fat. During a pre-breakfast morning workout, the body will burn more fat. You'll also have what is called the "afterburn" effect, which means that metabolism stays elevated for several hours even after your workout. Finally, working out in the morning gives you an endorphin rush and energy boost. This natural high can last for hours — even better than coffee!

Lift the right amount of weight

Building muscle helps you lose fat and drop unwanted pounds, but do you know how much is the right amount of weight to lift during strength training? If you lift weights that are too light, you won't see improvements in strength or muscle tone. If you lift weights that are too heavy, you'll compromise form and risk getting injured. You want to be able to perform 8 to 12 repetitions per set, choosing weights heavy enough that you struggle through your final few reps, but not so heavy that you sacrifice form. You should be maxed out by the last rep; if you feel like you could do another, increase the weight by 5 to 10 percent.

Another way to determine the weight you should be lifting is to find your "1 rep max" for an exercise (the weight at which you can only do one rep), then lift 60 to 80 percent of that amount.

Know how and when to eat to maximize your workouts

It's important to know which foods to eat before and after you exercise. Carbs that are low in fat give you the energy you need to have a great workout. Protein helps with muscle repair and growth. Fat also acts as fuel for workouts, although you should eat mostly unsaturated fats, such as those from nuts, avocados and fish.

Give yourself plenty of time for your body to digest a meal before working out, and specifically avoid fatty foods before exercising. Fats remain in your stomach longer, causing you to feel uncomfortable. However, having low blood sugar before a workout can cause dizziness and lethargy, so if you're famished, a small snack of peanut butter or low-fat cheese on whole wheat crackers can give you the boost you need to make it through an exercise session. After your workout, eating a meal packed with protein and carbohydrates within 2 hours can help replace energy-fueling glycogen stores.

During a pre-breakfast morning workout, the body will burn more fat. You'll also have what is called the "afterburn" effect, which means that metabolism stays elevated for several hours even after your workout.

Include interval training to torch calories and body fat

Your mission is to reduce your caloric intake or burn more calories through exercise than you take in a day. Interval training is a great way to blast through calories and body fat because it combines short bursts of intense activity with periods of lighter activity. As your cardiovascular fitness improves, you'll be able to go longer and up the intensity of the more difficult portions, helping you burn even more calories.

Here is one interval training workout that burns 500 or more calories in an hour. As your level of fitness improves, you should aim for a sprinting pace of at least 7.5 mph, a running pace of at least 6.0 mph, and a jogging pace of at least 5.0 mph. Your warm up and cool down paces can be slightly slower than a jog.

0:00–10:00 Warm up jog
10:00–10:20 Sprint
10:20–11:20 Jog
11:20–14:00 Repeat minutes
  10:00–11:20 twice
14:00–17:00 Jog
17:00–27:00 Run
27:00–31:00 Jog
31:00–35:00 Run
35:00–39:00 Jog
39:00–55:00 Repeat minutes
  31:00–39:00 twice
55:00–60:00 Gradually slow pace to
  jog/walk to cool down

Wear the right shoes

Just like getting new exercise clothes, having the right shoes improves your workout. Wearing the appropriate shoes for the activity — from running to weight lifting to basketball — also protects you from soreness and injury. For instance, running shoes are designed for forward heel-to-toe motion and do not provide the right ankle support for the side-to-side motion of activities like kickboxing or step aerobics. And not all running shoes provide the same cushioning and support. For instance, depending on whether you supinate (run on the outside of your feet) or overpronate (your feet roll inward as you run), you will need different types of running shoes. If you check out your old shoes, you should be able to see where the heel is worn down. Or, visit a specialty store to have your foot measured and your shoes professionally fit. A shoe should be snug but not be so tight that it puts pressure on the top of your foot or crushes your toes. And be sure to replace shoes every 300 to 500 miles, which you can monitor in your fitness journal.

> Wearing the appropriate shoes for the activity you choose — from running to weight lifting to basketball — protects you from soreness and injury.

Stay hydrated

Proper hydration is one of the easiest and most effective ways of boosting workout performance. Water is necessary in order for metabolism to take place, so being properly hydrated helps your body turn food into the energy you need for exercising. Water also helps your body regulate its temperature through sweating. Because vigorous exercise causes you to lose large amounts of water through sweating, it is important to drink water before, during, and after each workout session. Drink between 8 and 16 ounces of water in the hour prior to working out. Replenish fluids by drinking 4 to 8 ounces of water every 15 minutes during your workout. During vigorous cardiovascular training, or if you're exercising in hot temperatures, increase your water consumption in order to replace water lost from sweating. Then, drink between 8 and 16 ounces of water within 30 minutes of completing your exercise routine. Your muscles need water in order to recover from the stress of a workout. Drinking the right amounts of water after your workout will help reduce muscle soreness and help you feel less tired.

Hydrate right!

It's extremely important to stay fully hydrated before, during and after your workout — just don't reach for a sports drink that is full of unwanted calories. While slews of TV commercials featuring famous pro athletes lead you to believe that sports drinks like Gatorade and Vitamin Water help you stay fit and healthy, these drinks actually contain up to 200 calories and 35 grams of carbs per bottle. The promise that these drinks will give you the energy and electrolytes you need to have a great workout is really just a marketing ploy. For instance, Gatorade was originally developed to help college football players avoid dehydration and cramping during a rigorous training program in the humid summer months. A normal person like you, who is exercising at a much more moderate level, has no need for the carbs and calories in a sports drink. Water is always your best option. If you like the flavoring in sports drinks, try a low- or no-calorie version, like Powerade Zero or Gatorade's G2.

> Build one or two "light days" into your weekly workout schedule, but make them count! Light days might include biking, walking, dynamic stretching (walking lunges, trunk twists or arm circles, for instance), and swimming.

Don't overtrain

Want in on a fitness secret? There is such a thing as too much exercise. Let's say you're preparing to run a 5k race, and you start running several miles every day. You'll quickly notice that after a couple of weeks of training hard daily, your body begins to feel fatigued more quickly. Your muscles ache and you feel tired after just a short distance. You may find that you feel sore and even have trouble sleeping at night. These are all symptoms of overtraining. In order to lose up to 10 pounds in 2 weeks, you will need to do some form of exercise each day; however, you shouldn't aim for a high-intensity cardio or weight-lifting session every day. It's not realistic or good for your body, which needs periods of rest and recovery. Build one or two "light days" into your weekly workout schedule, but make them count! Schedule the same amount of time for your workout as a normal day, just exercise at a lower intensity. Light days might include biking, walking, dynamic stretching (walking lunges, trunk twists or arm circles, for instance), and swimming. Keep your body in motion but make sure you're giving hardworking muscles groups time to rest and recover so you're full of energy and stamina for your next tough workout.

Work toward your target heart rate

If you're not working out within your target heart rate zone, you're not getting the maximum benefits. The "fat burning zone," which burns the most calories and body fat stores, is reached at about 60 to 70 percent of your maximum heart rate. To calculate your maximum heart rate, subtract your age from 226 (for women, 220 for men). Then, multiply that number by 0.6 (60 percent) or 0.7 (70 percent) to find the number of beats

In addition to reps with weights, consider Power yoga, which can burn more than 400 calories per hour and works multiple muscle groups at once. Yoga is a great workout because you're lifting your own body weight in many poses.

per minute that is your target heart rate.

To determine whether you're in that zone during your workout, either wear a heart rate monitor or take your pulse for 10 seconds and multiply the number of beats by 6. Adjust your intensity depending on whether you are above or below your target heart rate.

Exercise muscles in proper progression to maximize results.

When you're working a variety of muscles during a strength-training sequence, order is important. If your workout includes a variety of weightlifting exercises, begin with your larger muscle groups and move to the smaller muscles. This allows for optimal performance of the most demanding exercises when your fatigue levels are at their lowest and you feel energized and fresh. The most important thing is to be sure that you have enough energy to complete your entire workout. It is better to do less and complete the entire circuit than to neglect a muscle group or do an uneven number of reps from one side of the body to the other.

As your level of fitness improves, you should up the intensity of your workouts. For example, when running, aim for a sprinting pace of at least 7.5 mph, a running pace of at least 6.0 mph, and a jogging pace of at least 5.0 mph.

Variety is the spice of life

Variety helps keep you happy and motivated in both your diet and your workouts. If you restrict your diet to the point that you're eating only fish and salad, for instance, you'll quickly lose interest and enthusiasm.

Variety also keeps your weight loss and calorie burning from plateauing. If you do the same exercises, at the same intensity, day after day, working out will get boring and your body will stop burning fat and calories as quickly. You'll find your weight loss comes to a standstill. You need to plan for workouts that work different muscle groups at different intensities throughout the week. Because you're trying to torch through unwanted pounds, you'll want to focus on cardio but also complement it with strength training.

In addition to reps with weights, consider Power yoga, which can burn more than 400 calories per hour and works multiple muscle groups at once. Yoga is such a great workout because you're lifting your own body weight in many poses. Whatever you choose to do, creating a varied workout schedule is imperative to losing 10 pounds.

Carbs that are low in fat give you the energy you need to have a great workout. Protein helps with muscle repair and growth. Fat also acts as fuel for workouts, although you should eat mostly unsaturated fats.

" Failure is not fatal, but failure to change might be. **"**

~ John Wooden

Chapter 14

Ultimate Fitness Tips

You're well on your way to a successful diet and fitness program and, by now, you're seeing the weight drop off, feeling healthier, and enjoying more energy than ever. To continue making progress, you need to keep your body from plateauing and your dedication from waning.

To round out your program, you need a few powerful secrets. In this chapter, learn how to exercise efficiently, stay inspired, and breeze through physical activity on a daily basis, without your workout feeling like "work."

Motivation, seeing results, and enjoyment are the keys to sticking with a fitness plan for 2 weeks, or any amount of time. This book has given you all the tools you need to lose up to 10 pounds faster than you ever thought possible — use this final fitness chapter to rev up your workouts and get the very most from every minute of physical activity you do.

Make a music playlist to stay motivated

Music has been proven to help people work out longer and with more energy, as well as providing a distraction from fatigue. Dr. Costas Karageorghis, who has studied the effects of music on physical performance for 20 years, says that a good workout song should be between 120 and 140 beats-per-minute, which corresponds to the average person's heart rate while doing moderate exercise (up the tempo if you're working out harder). Most pop, rap, heavy metal and many rock songs fall into this tempo range.

Even if it's not your favorite artist or a type of music that you'd listen to in your car, an upbeat song can help keep you going when your energy is low or you're nearing the end of a tough workout.

Work out with someone you see often, such as your neighbor, coworker, roommate or spouse, and you'll be best able to hold each other accountable.

Invest in new workout clothes

When you feel confident and have the proper exercise clothes, you will be more motivated to exercise, and you'll work out longer, too. Invest in a few new pieces of workout clothing and you'll be inspired and excited to wear them! Choose shirts, shorts, pants and sports bras in breathable, quick-drying fabrics that wick sweat away from the body. Exercise clothes should also stretch and move with you. Finally, be sure to get what you need for the specific activities you'll be doing, such as compression shorts for biking, form-fitting pants for yoga, and supportive undergarments for running.

Rehydrate and replenish with coconut water

Coconut water is one of the purest natural liquids around, second only to real water. It's one of nature's best superfoods! Unlike sugary sports drinks, coconut water contains natural electrolytes for energy and hydration but with minimal calories (typically about 60 per bottle). Coconut water has no added sugar and, with more potassium than a banana and 15 times more than most sports drinks, it prevents cramping and promotes muscle recovery during and after a workout. It also has myriad weight-loss benefits, such as increasing metabolism and promoting healthy thyroid function.

You can buy individual servings of coconut water at most health food stores and at many gyms and fitness studios. Its natural properties and benefits to your health and exercise program make it a favorite of cyclists, runners, trainers, yoginis, and more.

Use plyometrics to blast calories

Plyometrics are a great way to burn calories in a short amount of time. These types of exercise are designed to produce fast, powerful movements. The muscle is loaded and then contracted in rapid sequence. When these exercises are done in succession they burn calories quickly. Plyometrics are great because they are strength-building exercises that require endurance and cardiovascular stamina.

You can try mixing jump rope, jumping jacks, squat jumps, box jumps and other plyometric activities into your normal workouts, or refer to the *Lose Up to 10 Pounds in 2 Weeks* exercise plan chapter later in this book, which contains a complete, challenging plyometric workout.

Get Netflix

No one is recommending you sit on your couch with movies all night — but Netflix is actually a great, inexpensive way to work out at home! Their wide selection of exercise and fitness DVDs includes dance, aerobics, yoga, Pilates, strength training and more. Some DVDs are available for rental, delivered right to your mailbox and kept as long as you like, and others can be watched instantly online, or on a gaming console like Wii or Xbox. Workout DVDs are perfect for the times when you need a quick, 30-minute blast, don't have time to drive to the gym, or want to try something new in the privacy of your living room. Or, maybe you're not sure if Hollywood trainer Jillian Michaels' *30-Day Shred* is right for you? Netflix gives you the option to try specific exercise DVDs before buying them. Just be sure to type in the name of the video you want into the Search bar — the "Browse" feature shows only a very limited number of choices.

Find a fitness buddy

Losing weight and getting active are always easier with a partner, so invite a spouse or friend to join you in your weight-loss efforts, especially if he or she seems threatened by or uncomfortable with your weight loss. The great things about a workout buddy is he or she keeps you accountable, motivated on the days when you don't feel like exercising, and keeps you company on hikes, bike rides, and rock climbing trips. Plus, if you're just trying out a new form of exercise, such as surfing or kickboxing, having a partner can make it more fun and less scary. Make your workout buddy someone you see often, such as your neighbor, coworker, roommate or spouse, and you'll be best able to hold each other accountable. You'll have someone to celebrate with when you both drop 10 pounds!

Schedule a cardio session around a TV show or sporting event

Running or bicycling for an hour or more in a gym can get dull fast. One tip for getting through a longer cardio session is to plan it for a time when a favorite show, movie or sporting event is on TV. Time will fly by when you're watching the Lakers game or an hour-long sitcom. Just be sure to do this when you have at least 45 minutes or more of cardio and you can work at a steady pace and zone out a bit. You won't want to be distracted by the TV screen if you're trying to get through 30 minutes of interval training, for instance.

A good workout song should be between 120 and 140 beats-per-minute, which corresponds to the average person's heart rate while exercising.

Get a boost from pre-workout caffeine

The caffeine in natural sources such as coffee and green tea, or in pill form, benefits your workouts because it acts as a thermogenic. Themorgenics speed up your body's functions, including breath and heart rate, encouraging the body to use calories more quickly. Don't overdo it when it comes to caffeine, of course. Listen to your body, and if you feel lightheaded, dizzy or faint, stop what you're doing immediately, rest for a few minutes, and abstain from caffeine in the future. Otherwise, unless you're exercising at high altitudes or suffer from high blood pressure or another heart condition, taking 100 to 200 mg (one cup of coffee has about 100 mg) of caffeine

45 minutes before a workout can help you burn fat stores, speed up your metabolism, and help you power through a workout.

Count your steps with a pedometer

Start wearing a pedometer daily to measure how many steps you're taking and how many calories you're burning. Pedometers clip to your belt or pocket — or any spot where they will be perpendicular to the ground. They come in a variety of styles and price points — for less than $20 you can get a sleek, simple device that counts steps and calculates calories burned. Deluxe models play music, have audio features, and allow you to upload your daily stats into your computer to track your progress and meet goals. Many new mp3 players come with built-in pedometers, as well. You'll want to reference consumer reports that test the efficiency and accuracy of different makes and models.

Drinking several cups of green tea can boost your workout and burns about 70 extra calories per day.

For $99, a new Microsoft product called Fitbit accurately tracks your calories burned, steps taken, distance traveled and even sleep quality. On your Fitbit profile, you enter the calories you ate for the day and the data from your Fitbit device automatically calculates if you've met the distance and calorie goals you set for the day and week.

Blow off the gym!

Many people enjoy the routine schedule of going to the same location every day, but others find the gym stifling and somewhat limiting. Or, you may feel lost among the confusing machines, bustling trainers and intense gym rats. Be it burnout or pure intimidation, you may be looking for an alternative to the gym.

Naturally, getting outside in the fresh air is your best choice. If you live in a city where weather permits, add a fun activity to your weekly workout schedule — bike rides, hiking, surfing, horseback riding, rock climbing. Try something new to shake things up and stay motivated. Bootcamps are also a great way to burn hundreds of calories in a short amount of time. Beach or park bootcamps are popping up all over the country, as well as indoor sessions that combine strength training with cardio. Bootcamp use interval training — bursts of activity with short rests in between exercises — to blast calories and fat. Another gym alternative is joining a private yoga or Pilates studio. You'll get focused, professional instructors and classes without the overwhelming nature of a gym atmosphere.

Caffeine benefits your workouts because it acts as a thermogenic. Themorgenics speed up your body's functions, including breath and heart rate, encouraging the body to use calories more quickly.

There are really hundreds of exercises, classes and groups available. Check out the website MeetUp.com to find out what's going on in your area. From surfing moms to salsa dancing clubs, if you can imagine it, it's out there.

❝ It's not who you are that holds you back, it's who you think you're not. **❞**

~ Unknown

Chapter 15

Activities & Calories Burned

All types of physical activity burn calories. You don't have to slave away at a gym — normal daily activities, chores and errands also require your body to burn calories, in addition to exercise.

This chapter highlights some of the typical physical activities, from sports to household chores, that you can do to burn calories while losing 10 pounds. They range from light to moderate to vigorous, so incorporate something from each list every day, or combine activities.

Be aware that the exact number of calories you will burn for each activity varies based on your weight. The following list is an approximation for someone who weighs 150 pounds. If you weigh more, you will burn slightly more calories; if you weigh less than 150 pounds, you will burn slightly fewer calories. If you require an exact count, there are many websites that can estimate calories burned based on your weight, intensity of the workout, and the length of time you exercised.

Light Activities: 150 or Less Cal/Hr.

Billiards. 140

Lying down/sleeping 60

Office work. 140

Sitting 80

Standing 100

Moderate Activities: 150-350 Cal/Hr.

Aerobic dancing 340

Ballroom dancing 210

Bicycling (5 mph) 170

Bowling. 160

Canoeing (2.5 mph) 170

Dancing (social) 210

Gardening (moderate). 270

Golf (with cart). 180

Golf (without cart) 320

Grocery shopping 180

Horseback riding (sitting trot). 250

Light housework/cleaning, etc. 250

Pilates 240

Ping-pong 270

Surfing 300

Swimming (20 yards/min). 290

Tennis (recreational doubles). 310

Vacuuming 220

Volleyball (recreational) 260

Walking (2 mph). 200

Walking (3 mph). 240

Walking (4 mph). 300

Vigorous Activities: 350 or More Cal/Hr.

Aerobics (step)......................................440

Backpacking (10 lb load)......................540

Badminton 450

Basketball (competitive) 660

Basketball (leisure) 390

Bicycling (10 mph)..............................375

Bicycling (13 mph) 600

Cross country skiing (leisurely)............460

Cross country skiing (moderate)..........660

Hiking 460

Ice skating (9 mph) 384

Jogging (5 mph)..................................550

Jogging (6 mph) 690

Racquetball..620

Rock Climbing 740

Rollerblading 384

Rowing machine..................................540

Running (8 mph)..................................900

Scuba diving 570

Shoveling snow 580

Soccer..580

Spinning 650

Stair climber machine 480

Swimming (50 yards/min.) 680

Water aerobics....................................400

Water skiing 480

Weight training (30 sec. between sets)....760

Weight training (60 sec. between sets)....570

Yoga (Power).......................................400

❝The greatest wealth is health.❞

~ Virgil

Chapter 16

Lose Up to 10 Pounds in 2 Weeks
Exercise Plan

No Exercise Equipment Required!

Losing weight requires a fitness plan full of high-intensity, calorie-blasting exercises that work the whole body. The *Lose Up to 10 Pounds in 2 Weeks* exercise plan is designed to target multiple muscle groups, build core strength, and get the heart rate elevated to burn body fat.

Six days out of each week you will pair a strength training circuit with a cardio circuit. You won't need any props or weights — just water to drink, stable exercise shoes, and moveable, breathable workout clothing. You will switch off each day between an upper body and core strength training circuit and a lower body and core strength training circuit. You will also alternate between a plyometric cardio circuit and a kickboxing cardio circuit. The last day of the week is to rest.

Every strength training exercise comes with step-by-step instructions, as well as modifications to make the move easier or harder. You may want to challenge yourself more on some exercises, or modify some moves to avoid injury or account for soreness.

For the cardio circuits, you will be able to work faster and harder without sacrificing form as your fitness level improves.

How to Do the Exercise Plan

You will need to set aside about 60 minutes to complete this workout plan. Do each exercise for 50 seconds, as many reps as you can do in that time without sacrificing form. Take a 10-second rest to get ready for the next exercise. Keep your eye on a stopwatch, timer on an mp3 player, or clock with a seconds hand. Complete all 6 exercises in the strength training circuit, then repeat the full circuit for a second round, and again for a third round. After you have completed 3 rounds of the strength training circuit, take a 2-minute water break and move on to the cardio circuit. Do the same for the cardio circuit.

Warming Up and Cooling Down

Always begin and end your strength training and cardio workouts with a 5- to 10-minute warm-up and cool-down. Walk, lightly jog or run in place to loosen the muscles. Next, stretch to prepare your muscles for work and prevent injury.

Important stretches include holding the heel close to the glute to stretch the quad muscle, reaching toward the toes to stretch hamstrings, calf stretches against a wall, and stretching your arms behind your head and across the chest to loosen shoulders, chest, biceps and triceps.

The same routine after your workout will bring the heart rate down, help the body recover and prevent soreness.

Your Workout Schedule

You only have 2 short weeks to get the body you've always wanted, so work hard and push yourself, even if it's to do one more rep! You'll love the feeling of success and pride you'll get after a tough workout. The body, strength and shape you've always wanted is just a couple of weeks away.

WEEK 1	STRENGTH	CARDIO
Mon	Upper Body & Core	Plyometrics
Tues	Lower Body & Core	Kickboxing
Wed	Upper Body & Core	Plyometrics
Thurs	Lower Body & Core	Kickboxing
Fri	Upper Body & Core	Plyometrics
Sat	Lower Body & Core	Kickboxing
Sun	Rest Day!	Rest Day!

WEEK 2	STRENGTH	CARDIO
Mon	Upper Body & Core	Kickboxing
Tues	Lower Body & Core	Plyometrics
Wed	Upper Body & Core	Kickboxing
Thurs	Lower Body & Core	Plyometrics
Fri	Upper Body & Core	Kickboxing
Sat	Lower Body & Core	Plyometrics
Sun	Rest Day!	Rest Day!

Notes:

_____

_____

_____

_____

_____

_____

_____

_____

_____

_____

_____

_____

_____

_____

_____

_____

_____

_____

_____

_____

_____

_____

_____

_____

_____

_____

_____

_____

STRENGTH TRAINING
UPPER BODY & CORE
CHEST, ARMS, SHOULDERS, BACK & CORE

Strength training is a very important part of losing weight. It lengthens and tones your body while replacing body fat with muscle, which burns three times as many calories as fat.

The exercises in this section work the upper body, including the chest, arms, shoulders, back and core. When coupled with the cardio programs described later in this chapter, you will get in shape quickly. Plus, they're fun and challenging!

JUDO PUSHUPS

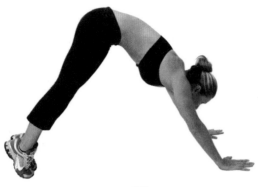

❶ Put your hands and feet on the ground with hips lifted so your body forms an inverted V shape.

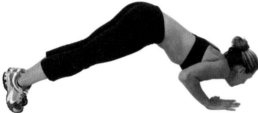

❷ Keeping your hips up, bend your arms out to the side, and lower your upper body until your chin is near the floor.

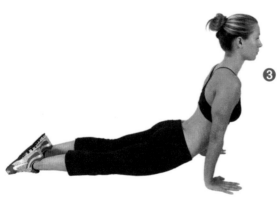

❸ Lower your hips toward the floor while you lift your upper body simultaneously. Then slide back into the original position, reversing the way you went in, for one rep.

Make It Easier: Put your knees on the ground as you lower your hips to the floor.

Make It Harder: Lift one leg.

BURPEES

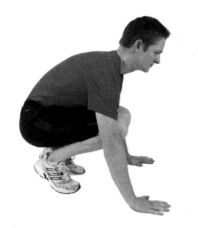

❶ Begin standing. Drop into a squat position with hands on the floor in front of you.

❷ Kick your feet back into a pushup position without letting your hips sag.

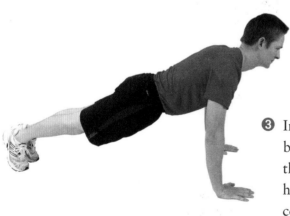

❸ Immediately jump your feet back to the squat position; then jump straight up as high as you can for one complete rep.

Make It Easier: Walk your feet back into pushup position.

Make It Harder: Move as quickly as you can through the reps. Jump as high as you can each time.

SIDE PLANK W/ PUSHUP

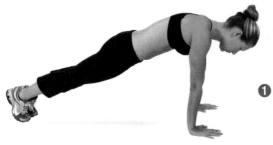

❶ Start in plank position.

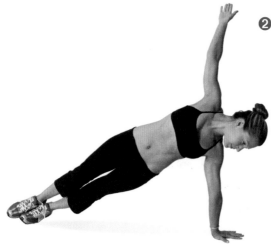

❷ Flip to one side; straighten your bottom arm directly under your shoulder, legs straight, and feet stacked. Place your free hand on your hip or stretch it up. Keep your back straight and do not allow your hips to sag. Work on tightening your abs and lifting your side away from the ground.

❸ Flip back to plank and complete a pushup.

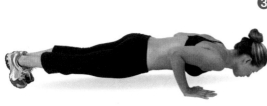

Make It Easier: Place one knee on the ground when you flip to the side.

Make It Harder: Lift the top leg up in side plank.

ARMS DIPS

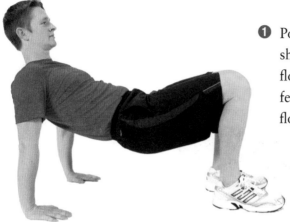

❶ Position your hands shoulder-width apart on the floor behind you and place feet hip-width apart on the floor in front of you.

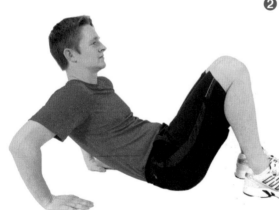

❷ Lift your hips so you are in a crab-like position. Bend your elbows and lower your hips down toward the floor. Then, press into your hands back up to your starting position. Don't straighten your arms all the way; keep your elbows slightly bent to keep tension on the arm muscles.

Make It Easier: Move your feet closer to your body.

Make It Harder: Straighten your legs out in front of you.

BENT KNEE V-UP

❶ Lie on the floor with arms straight alongside the body and legs out straight.

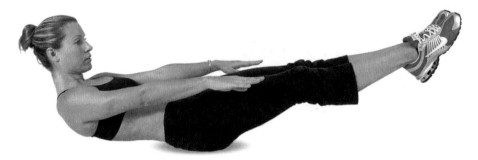

❷ Simultaneously, lift your chest and bring your knees toward the chest in a crunch. Lower back toward the starting position for one rep.

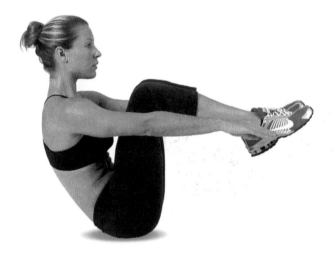

Make It Easier: Keep the back and shoulders on the ground and bring knees up into the body.

Make It Harder: Do a V Up by simultaneously lifting your arms and legs straight up in a V shape as if trying to touch your toes at the top.

REACHING PLANK

1 Position yourself face down and prop yourself up on your elbows, forearms, and toes in a plank position. Maintain a flat back and tighten your abs so the hips don't sag.

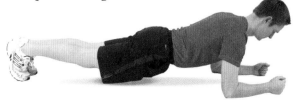

2 Next, inhale and lift one leg, lengthening and holding for a few seconds.

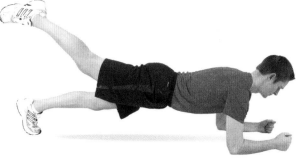

3 Return to plank, and reach out in front of your body with your opposite hand. Switch and perform on the other leg.

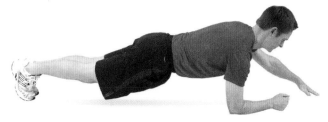

Make It Easier: Skip the reach. Or, bend knees and place them on the ground.

Make It Harder: Lift the leg higher and squeeze the glutes. Don't let your hips sag.

Notes:

STRENGTH TRAINING
LOWER BODY
LEGS, GLUTES & CORE

These lower body exercises will whip your legs, glutes and core into shape in just 2 weeks. You'll feel leaner, stronger and more explosive, especially when you combine these moves with the cardio exercises described later in this chapter.

Don't forget to challenge yourself as much as possible, and modify as necessary to push yourself or account for injuries or sore muscles.

WIDE SQUATS

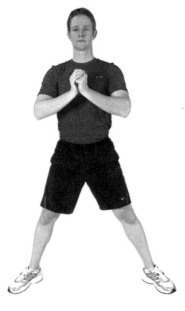

❶ Stand with feet wide, toes turned out slightly, with hands together at chest height.

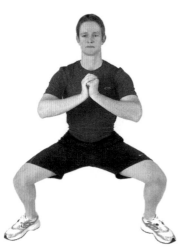

❷ Squat low to the ground, squeezing the glutes. As you come up, lift your arms over your head until they are straight, for one complete rep. Be sure to keep the core engaged and don't hunch forward. Push through the feet to rise up and return to starting position.

Make It Easier: Don't sink as low to the ground.

Make It Harder: Go slowly, and focus the weight into your heels.

LUNGES WITH A TWIST

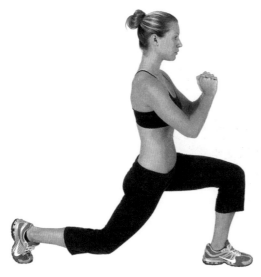

❶ Start standing, then step forward into a lunge, making sure your knee doesn't go past your toes.

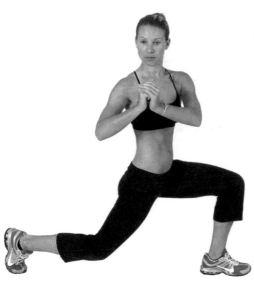

❷ When you reach the lowest point of your lunge, twist your torso to the side, squeezing the core. Stand up from the lunge and repeat on the other leg. Keep your back straight and your thigh parallel to the ground in your lunge.

Make It Easier: Don't sink as low in your lunge.

Make It Harder: Twist and lunge slowly and more deeply.

BRIDGE POSE

❶ Lie flat with knees bent and hip-width apart; tuck your pelvis so your lower back touches the floor.

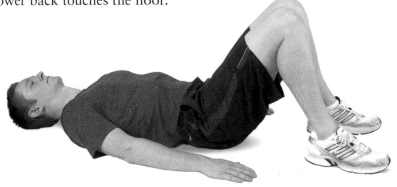

❷ Raise your hips until your body forms a straight line from shoulders to knees. Squeeze your glutes, engage abs, and elevate through the thighs. Hold for 2 to 5 seconds and lower to the floor.

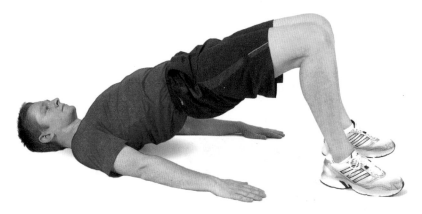

Make It Easier: Move your feet away from your body.

Make It Harder: Pull your feet as close to your body as you can. Lift one leg and hold for a few seconds. Lower and lift the other leg before returning to start position.

BICYCLES

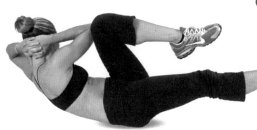

❶ Lie on your back with your knees bent at a 90-degree angle.

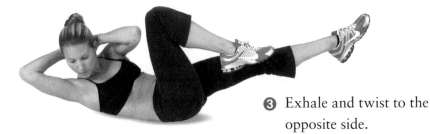

❷ Lace your fingers behind your head. Lift your head and shoulders, exhale and twist to one side, bringing your knee in toward your opposite elbow, while straightening the other leg. Return to center, inhale.

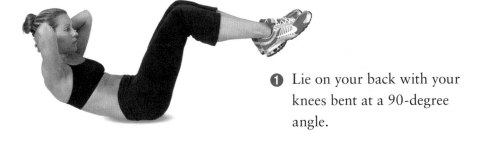

❸ Exhale and twist to the opposite side.

Make It Easier: Keep feet on the ground and slide heels along the floor using a towel.

Make It Harder: Perform bicycles as fast as you can, being sure to rotate from the core.

FIRE HYDRANT

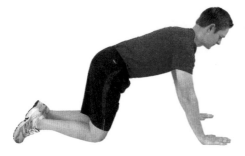

❶ Get on the floor on your hands and knees with a flat back, in a table position.

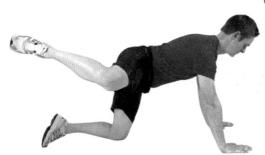

❷ Keeping your knee bent, lift one knee up and out to the side. Try to lift the knee as high as your hip, or whatever height is comfortable, squeezing the glutes.

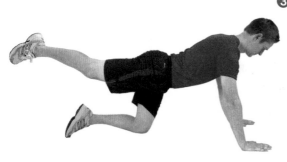

❸ Next, kick the raised leg back until it is straight behind you. Lower the leg to the starting position and repeat, switching legs at the 25-second mark.

Make It Easier: Skip the kick back.

Make It Harder: Raise the leg higher, squeezing the glutes.

RUSSIAN TWIST

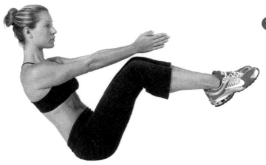

❶ Sit with your legs bent. Hold arms out in front of you and press the palms together. Lean slightly back so your upper body forms a 45-degree angle with the floor and lift your feet off the floor.

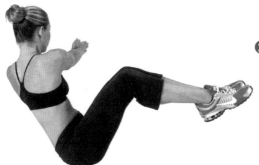

❷ Rotate your arms with palms pressed as far to one side as you can, reaching over while you squeeze your abs and obliques.

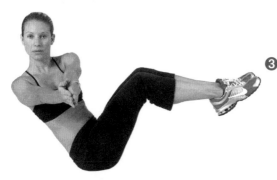

❸ Return to center and twist to the other side. Keep your feet lifted and centered; rotate from your core, not your hips.

Make It Easier: Keep your feet flat on the ground.

Make It Harder: Cycle your legs as you twist. When you twist to the right, extend your left leg and pull your right knee into your chest; repeat on the other side. Don't let your feet touch the floor at any point.

Notes:

CARDIO
PLYOMETRICS

Plyometrics are a great way to build muscle, burn a lot of calories in a short amount of time, and get your heart rate up. During all plyometric exercises it is important to keep knees slightly bent when pushing off and landing. Never land with a thud; think of exploding out, using your muscles to coil and spring. Be sure to stretch well and warm up and cool down before and after this circuit.

JUMPING JACKS

❶ Stand with feet together and arms by your sides.

❷ Jump legs out to the sides, simultaneously raising arms overhead; then immediately jump back to the starting position. Repeat as fast as you can, focusing on controlling the arms and legs.

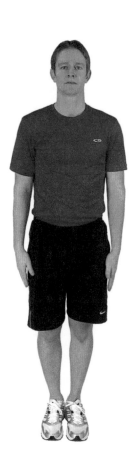

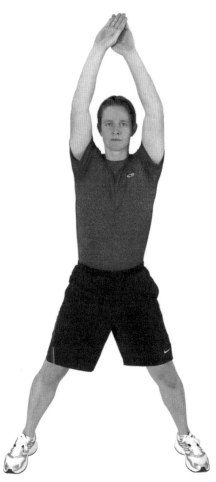

SPLIT JUMPS

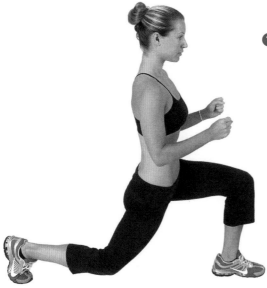

❶ Start in a low lunge stance.

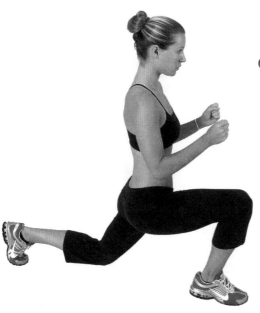

❷ Bend the knees and jump, switching legs to land in the same position on the opposite leg. Go as quickly as you can without sacrificing form.

HIGH KNEES

❶ Bend your arms at 90-degree angles and hold them out in front of you, palms down.

❷ Start running in place, lifting the knees as high as your palms. Running on the toes will make this exercise more beneficial. Make sure you don't lean too far back. Repeat as fast as you can.

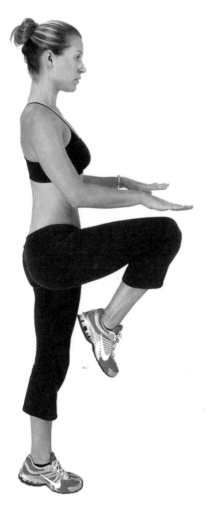

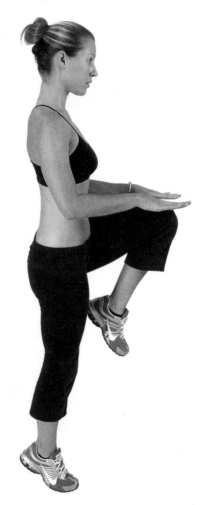

STAR JUMP

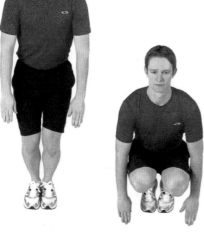

❶ Stand with your knees slightly bent.

❷ Squat down and get ready to explode out.

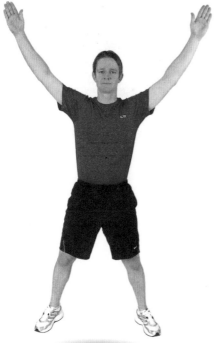

❸ Jump as high as you can, stretching your arms and legs out to the sides in a star shape in the air. Before you land, pull your arms and legs back to your body, landing in the starting position. Repeat with little to no rest between jumps.

LATERAL JUMP

❶ Choose a low, flat object you can jump over, such as a broomstick or jump rope. Start standing on one side.

❷ Jump sideways to opposite side of the object, then immediately jump back to other side and repeat as quickly as possible.

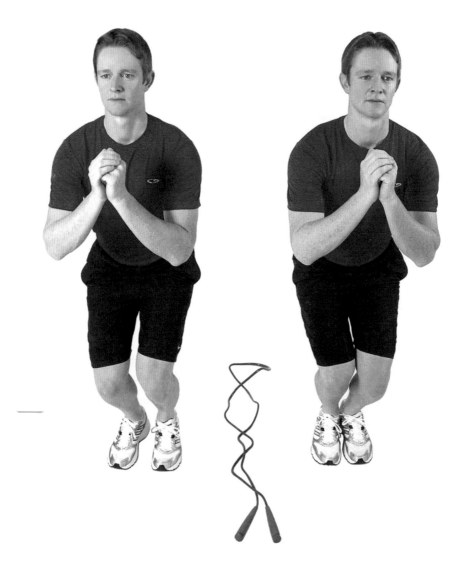

MOUNTAIN CLIMBERS

❶ Begin in a pushup position with arms straight. Bring one knee in toward the chest, placing the toe on the floor.

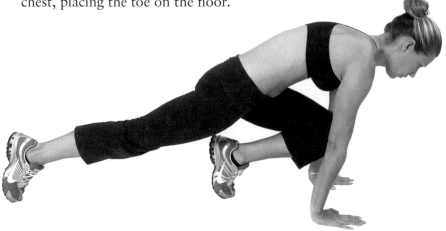

❷ Jump and switch legs in the air, bringing the back foot in and the front foot back. Continue alternating the feet as fast as you can without sacrificing form.

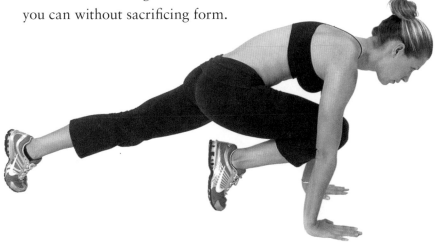

Notes:

KICKBOXING

This fast fat-burning workout is fun and dynamic, and it improves cardio conditioning and increases endurance. It can be done anywhere, just be sure you have ample room for kicks and jabs at full extension. Keep abs engaged throughout the entire sequence and don't sacrifice form for speed. Inhale before you kick or jab and exhale during the kick or jab.

Be sure to walk for a few minutes or jog in place to warm up the body for this cardio plan.

FRONT KICK

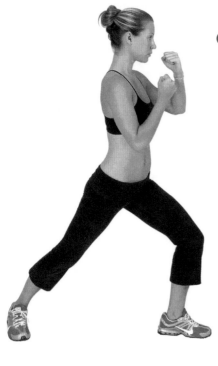

1 Stand with left foot forward in fighting stance, fists up. Begin to shift your weight to the left foot.

2 Kick straight out as if you were reaching with the ball of the foot. Retract immediately and return to fighting stance. Do as many kicks with the right leg as you can and switch to the left leg halfway through at the 25-second mark.

UPPERCUT

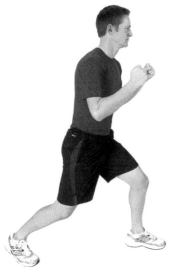

1 Start in fighting stance, holding your arms with elbows bent and close to your body.

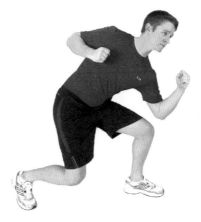

2 Get low for power, and step into the punch, pushing your left fist up. Remember to push through your legs.

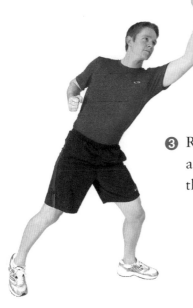

3 Recoil and repeat, switching arms halfway through, at the 25-second mark.

KNEE KICK

❶ Begin in fighting stance, with the kicking leg back. Reach up with your arms, as if pulling an imaginary opponent toward you, and drive your knee up, keeping your toes pointed down. Bend your bottom leg slightly for leverage.

❷ Drop the kicking leg back down, and repeat, alternating legs halfway through at the 25-second mark.

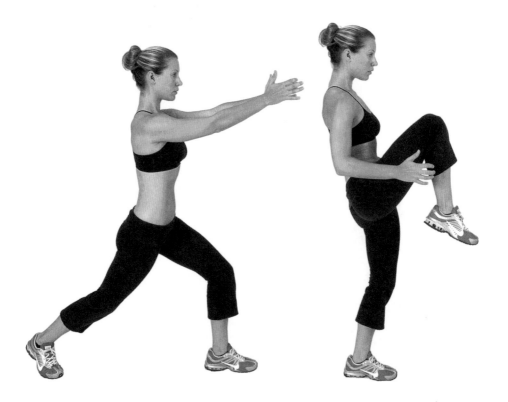

SIDE KICK

1 Start in a horse stance, with feet slightly wider than shoulder-width apart, feet pointing forward, and knees slightly bent and out to the side.

2 Lift your right knee toward your chest, keeping your foot flexed.

3 Kick your right leg out to the side, pushing through the heel while counterbalancing by bending your upper body slightly toward the left. Retract the kick and immediately return to horse stance.

Practice keeping your fists near your face. Alternate the kicking leg.

RIGHT & LEFT PUNCH

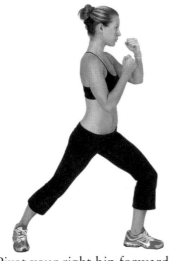

❶ Stand with left foot forward in fighting stance, with fists up.

❷ Pivot your right hip forward, extending and jabbing with the right arm. Your fist should be parallel to the floor at full extension, and your arm should be in line with your shoulder.

❸ Recoil immediately and punch with the left arm, pulling the right arm back, close to the body. Repeat as fast as you can without sacrificing form, switching legs at the 25-second mark.

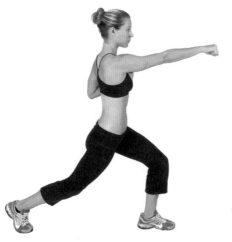

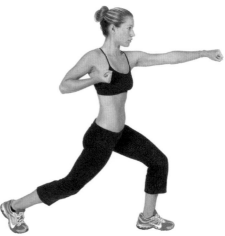

BACK KICK

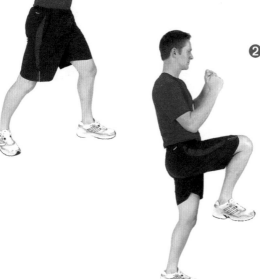

❶ Stand in fighting stance.

❷ Placing your weight down into the front leg, lift the right knee, then kick back through that leg, flexing your foot and using the heel as a striking surface.

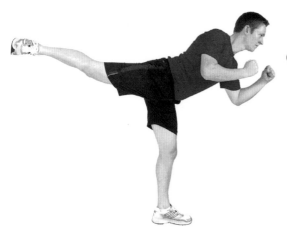

❸ Lower your leg back to the starting position. Do as many kicks with the right leg as you can and switch to the left leg halfway through at the 25-second mark.

"Whether you think you can or think you can't
— you are right.**"**

~ Henry Ford

Secrets to Get Fit
At-A-Glance

The program outlined in this book is packed with information, tips, and practical knowledge that, when implemented daily, will help you lose more weight and get in better shape than you ever imagined, in just 14 days.

Refer to the following section, which contains 100 fast fitness secrets, when you need a reminder, inspiration, or motivation to stay active and eat right every day. Not only will these tips be useful throughout this program, they'll be effective after the 2 weeks, as at-a-glance reminders of the benefits of being physically fit and sticking with a healthy eating plan.

Don't forget — healthy weight loss can never be achieved with fitness alone, so combine an active lifestyle with eating the right foods in the right amounts. You'll be amazed at how you look and feel!

SECRETS TO GET FIT AT-A-GLANCE

1. **Counteract the effects of aging with physical activity.** Exercising decreases the chance of developing arthritis or osteoporosis by increasing muscle tone and bone density. Additionally, increased circulation supports the production of collagen, which fights wrinkles.

2. **Exercise to decrease your risk of heart disease.** Exercise strengthens the heart muscle and helps reduce cholesterol in the blood, so exercise daily to combat heart disease.

3. **Increase lean muscle mass to burn more fat.** Studies have shown that for every pound of muscle you add to your body, you will burn an additional 35 to 50 calories per day!

4. **Enjoy more consistent and restful sleep when you exercise.** Studies have shown that if the body remains too sedentary during its active phase, it may have a difficult transition into sleep. Build up intensity with exercise and sleep more deeply.

5. **Exercise to decrease depression and anxiety.** Get moving! Research suggests that exercising 30 minutes a day, 3 to 5 days a week, can significantly improve the symptoms of depression.

6. **Enjoy newfound self-confidence.** Sticking to a diet and fitness plan and meeting your goals has a collateral effect in the form of greater self-esteem, which will help improve other aspects of your life, such as your professional and social life.

7. **Exercise to improve your social life.** A healthy, active lifestyle is filled with opportunities for meeting others who care about health, from social encounters at the gym, an activities group, or a fitness class.

8. **Get your body in motion and it will want to remain in motion.** Your body not only needs exercise to function well, it actually craves it. With every workout session, your desire to be physically active will naturally increase.

9. **Enjoy social interactions while you exercise.** Being social with people while you get in shape makes you look forward to working out and makes you stay at the gym longer.

10. **Exercise to help you quit smoking.** Quitting smoking? Benefits of exercise include fewer withdrawal symptoms, such as irritability, restlessness, tension, and poor concentration. Plus, the desire to light up can be delayed 2 or 3 times longer for people who exercise.

11. **Clear your head and increase brain function with exercise.** When you exercise, it increases not only your blood circulation but also the oxygen and glucose that reach your brain. More blood flow enhances your energy production and waste removal.

12. **Lower your blood pressure with regular exercise.** As your heart grows stronger in response to exercise, it can pump more blood with less force, and your blood pressure goes down.

13. **Set realistic, challenging goals.** To avoid giving up on your workout program, set goals that are difficult, but achievable. You should be challenged, but you should have opportunities for success.

14. **Start the day with exercise.** Wake up your body by working out in the morning and getting much-needed oxygen to your muscles and brain. Your metabolism will remain at the higher

level, and you will continue to burn calories at a higher rate, even hours after you've worked out.

15. **Use visualization to improve results.** Visualize the specific aspects of your workout. Picture the energy surging through you as you hike a steep trail. Imagine your abs lengthening and tightening as you perform core exercises.

16. **Do not compare yourself to others.** We all have different fitness potential and body composition. Instead of measuring your success as it compares to others, measure it by the amount of effort you put forth and your physical improvements.

17. **Plan your workouts ahead of time.** Block out time for your workouts on a calendar days or weeks in advance. Make time for working out instead of working out if you have the time.

18. **Make realistic changes to accommodate your workout program.** Look for opportunities to fit exercise into your existing lifestyle. If you are not a morning person, it is probably unrealistic to plan to wake up and exercise before work. Instead, try working out in the early evening or on your lunch hour.

19. **Personalize your fitness routine by choosing activities you enjoy.** Working out shouldn't be work. It shouldn't be boring. Choose activities that stimulate you mentally and challenge you physically, and you are going to be far more likely to stick with your fitness plan.

20. **Diversify your workouts to avoid boredom and improve results.** Mix up your cardio and strength-training regimen with a weekly Pilates class or rock climbing class. Diversifying your workout keeps you from becoming bored and works different

muscles all the time.

21. **Plan to work out with a partner so you won't skip out.** Workout partners are a built-in backup plan to help you maintain your exercise schedule. Choose a neighbor, roommate, or coworker; if your partner is someone you see on a regular basis, you are more likely to stay committed.

22. **Replace self-doubt with positive thoughts.** Henry Ford, founder of Ford Motor Company, once said, "If you think you can do a thing or think you can't do a thing, you're right." Replace your negative thoughts with positive ones.

23. **Use visual aids to set goals, motivate, and show success.** Even something as simple as placing a sticker or smiley face in your fitness journal on the days you worked out can help motivate you to exercise more regularly.

24. **Celebrate your achievements.** Reward yourself but keep in line with your healthy lifestyle. If you lost 4 pounds, for example, don't celebrate with a high-calorie meal. A more appropriate reward might be a new article of clothing.

25. **Measure your weight properly.** To get an accurate measurement, weigh yourself as soon as you wake up in the morning, without clothes, before eating or drinking anything.

26. **Use cardiovascular exercise to improve how the heart works.** Repetitious exercise with brief moments of rest force your heart to improve its ability to pump oxygen and blood. Activities such as running, walking, swimming, and bicycling are all excellent for cardiovascular training and will get noticeable easier as you do them.

27. **Use the Talk Test to determine your cardio workout intensity.** Gauge your workout intensity with the Talk Test. Work out at a level at which you can answer questions, but not carry on a conversation.

28. **Know your target heart rate to improve your workout efficiency.** Work out at 60 to 70 percent of your maximum heart rate (MHR) for full fat-burning results. To determine your MHR, subtract your age from 220, then multiply by .60 or .70 to find your target heart rate.

29. **Spend at least 20 minutes on aerobic exercise to begin to burn stored fat.** It typically takes 20 minutes of steady aerobic exercise before your body begins to draw on its fat supply.

30. **Vary your cardiovascular activities so you don't plateau.** Your body will respond by growing stronger when it is forced to work in new ways and you will find that switching your routine will invigorate you.

31. **Increase your HDL and lower your LDL cholesterol with strength training.** Recent studies have shown convincing links between strength training and increased HDL cholesterol in the body's arteries. Healthy cholesterol levels significantly lower your risk of heart disease.

32. **Use household items to strength train.** You don't need a gym or fancy equipment for strength training. Use 1-gallon bottles of bleach and 1- and 5-pound bags of pasta, rice, or beans for arms. Squat and lunge with a 10-pound bag of dog food to work legs.

33. **Perfect your form for the best results.** Strength training

relies on the isolation and overloading of specific muscles, so it is essential to learn proper technique. Meet with a personal trainer who can show you the best way to perform exercises and use strength training machines.

34. **Increase your muscle mass by increasing weight and decreasing repetitions.** When you are training for strength, lift at 80 to 90 percent of your maximum weight, decrease your reps, and increase the time between sets slightly.

35. **Decrease weight and increase repetitions for more muscle definition.** To create long lean muscles, train at around 60 to 70 percent of maximum intensity for 15 to 20 repetitions per set.

36. **Increase muscular endurance by decreasing rest time between sets.** Muscular endurance is important for doing an activity for a long period of time. Drop down to 40 to 60 percent of your maximum intensity and increase your repetitions to 20 or more.

37. **Use your body weight to develop strength.** You have an amazing strength-training tool for fitness and endurance training right in your own body weight! Typical body weight exercises include pushups, sit-ups, pull-ups, and dips.

38. **Begin and end every workout session with stretching.** Warm-up stretches before you exercise prepare the body for work by increasing blood flow to the muscles and by relieving tension in the muscles. A proper cool down will also help reduce muscle soreness.

39. **Use flexibility training to prevent injury.** Increased

flexibility strengthens tendons, ligaments, and muscles. Stronger tendons and ligaments protect your muscles and help prevent them from becoming strained or knotted.

40. **Use passive stretching and deliberate breathing to target specific muscles.** During passive stretching, concentrate on slow, deep breaths through the nose to relieve tension as you move further into each stretch.

41. **Try yoga as a fun and effective method of flexibility training.** In addition to greatly improving flexibility, yoga creates better posture, increased stamina, increased energy, improved balance, and injury prevention and recovery. Yoga classes are available at gyms and private studios for every age and skill level.

42. **Hold stretches longer as you get older.** Muscles become less pliable as we age, so if you're over 40, hold each stretch for 60 seconds. If you're under 40, you can hold stretches for 30 seconds.

43. **Avoid bouncing when stretching.** Bouncing during stretching, such as bouncing while you reach for your toes, can lead to injury. Try bending your knees slightly to reach your toes, rather than bouncing.

44. **Consult a doctor about taking a daily multivitamin or mineral supplement.** Vitamins and minerals are substances your body needs in small but steady amounts for normal growth, function, and health. Ask your doctor which ones might be right to boost your fitness program.

45. **Massage muscles to help them warm up for flexibility training.** Massage increases blood flow and improves circulation,

relaxes muscles, prevents painful cramps, and helps remove waste products, such as lactic acid, which prevents post-exercise soreness.

46. **Maximize your fitness performance through proper hydration.** Just a 2 percent loss in water supply can lead to a 20 percent decrease in energy levels. Drink lots of water before, during and after your workouts to maximize fitness performance.

47. **Compensate for caffeine.** Adjust water consumption to compensate for fluid loss if you drink caffeinated coffee, soda or tea. A simple way to ensure that you are drinking enough water is to drink a full cup of water each time you refill your coffee mug.

48. **Avoid dehydration by drinking water before you feel thirsty.** It can take more than an hour for the effects of dehydration to be felt in your body. Drink water throughout the day to avoid dehydration.

49. **Burn 3,500 excess calories to lose 1 pound.** To lose weight, you must create a calorie deficit where your body uses more calories than you consume. It takes approximately 3,500 excess calories to gain a pound; conversely, you must burn about 3,500 calories to lose a pound.

50. **Burn calories through everyday activities.** Burn extra calories any place you can, including shopping, cleaning, gardening, and walking the dog. Every extra step counts.

51. **Eat complex carbohydrates to raise your metabolism.** Complex carbohydrates help you burn more calories, which results in accelerated weight loss. Complex carbs can be found in whole

grain bread, cereal, rice, pasta, tortillas, crackers, beans, yams, peas, and more.

52. **Feel full longer and build lean muscle mass when you eat lean protein.** Try to include 1 serving of a lean, protein-rich food, such as skinless poultry, fish, egg whites, low-fat or fat-free milk products, beans, nuts, or tofu, with every meal.

53. **Maintain steady blood-sugar levels to enhance cardiovascular training.** Select slow-burning carbohydrates, such as potatoes, oatmeal, and brown rice, so that you are able to maintain blood sugar at a steady level. Avoid sugar because it leads to energy crashes in the middle of a workout session.

54. **Replenish your body with nutrients quickly after workout sessions.** The proper post-workout meal of carbohydrate- and protein-rich foods with very little fat boosts your metabolism and strengthens and heals muscles.

55. **Know both the risks and benefits of taking exercise supplements.** While exercise supplements may provide improved endurance, concentration, and coordination in the short-term, the long-term benefits and problems have not been fully researched. Do not take energy and performance enhancers without first consulting your doctor.

56. **Stay fit while on vacation.** A massage or lounging by the pool are nice, but they won't keep you fit. Vacation in a spot where you can hike, bike, ride horses, whitewater raft, kayak, or try other adventurous fitness activities.

57. **Avoid crash diets, which slow your basal metabolic**

rate. Your BMR, or the amount of calories burned when the body is at rest, slows down if you go on an intensely restrictive diet as the body prepares to go into starvation mode. Healthy eating and a regular fitness schedule keep your BMR active.

58. **Don't skip meals if you want to lose weight.** Skipping meals not only causes your metabolism to slow down, it means you won't have enough energy to complete your workouts. Don't make the mistake of skipping regular meals.

59. **Use potassium to recover from workouts.** Potassium helps your muscles heal after a tough workout. Bananas, sweet potatoes, yogurt, tomato juice, coconut water, and spinach are all great sources of potassium.

60. **Fuel workouts with monounsaturated and polyunsaturated fats.** Fat is critical to a healthy diet and is an excellent source of fuel for your workouts. Sources of good fats include salmon, olives, avocados, and nuts. Limit saturated fats, which your body can't burn as fuel.

61. **Reach your goals with a personal trainer.** A trainer will teach you proper technique and use of machines, will help to motivate you through difficult times, and will also help you maximize your workout sessions.

62. **Learn something new in a group exercise class.** From bootcamps to kickboxing to aerobics, group classes usually include a combo of cardio, strength, and flexibility training. Ask for a schedule of classes at your local gym or look online for a private studio in your area.

63. **Use music as an excellent motivator.** Listening to music can motivate you to relieve stress and push yourself further during your workouts. Download faster songs with 120 beats per minute or more to get you moving.

64. **Stretch at your desk.** Sit tall in your chair, stretch both arms over your head, and reach as high as you can for 10 seconds. For your neck, roll your head gently to each side, so that your ear almost touches your shoulder. Hold for 10 seconds.

65. **Use every chance you get to get up and walk around.** Desk jobs leave people sedentary for hours on end. Pace while talking on the phone or walk over to a colleague's desk instead of sending an email.

66. **Get fit as a family.** Find activities your family can do together so you never use time with them as a reason for passing on exercise. Try yoga, bike riding, surfing, or tossing a football. For very young children, a game of tag is enough to get everyone moving.

67. **Use a pedometer or heart monitor to track your workout.** Using a pedometer allows you to track the number of steps you take and encourages you to walk and run further each day. Try to take about 10,000 steps a day.

68. **Learn proper mechanics of gym and fitness equipment.** When using equipment for the first time, read the instructions on the side of the machine and go slowly in order to avoid injury. Don't be afraid to ask gym employees to explain how a piece of fitness equipment works.

69. **Know your limitations.** Pace yourself and work with a partner

or spotter when training with heavy free weights. Avoid pushing yourself too hard at the start of a fitness routine.

70. **Stop making excuses and find solutions instead.**
In order to better prepare yourself for the excuses to skip exercise that will inevitably come up, write them down, then write down how you plan to overcome them.

71. **Protect your neck during core exercises.** Situps have their merit but can put strain on neck muscles. Lace your fingers together and put your hands behind your head; then, keep your neck properly aligned and crunch with your abs, not your head.

72. **Allow 2 days rest between strength-training sessions.** Resting is an essential part of strength training so that your muscles have time to rest and heal. Give muscle groups 2 days between sessions.

73. **Stop working out if you feel dizzy, in pain or faint.** If you are working out and feel sharp pain or dizziness, stop, sit down, and drink water until you feel well enough to head home. Don't try to push through pain or illness.

74. **Don't exercise if you're sick.** Give yourself a day off from exercise if you're feeling sick, or have a fever or cough. The lungs and heart are forced to work harder when you're sick and a workout can dangerously exacerbate that.

75. **Consider an online personal trainer.** A low-cost alternative to hiring a personal trainer is to use one that you find online. These trainers will help you select appropriate exercise routines for your lifestyle and fitness goals and will track your results via

email or text messaging.

76. **Invest in quality exercise shoes.** Select shoes with the best support and cushioning for the activities you're doing. While at the store, you should walk around, run in place, and jump to check the fit.

77. **Understand that setbacks are not failures.** Allow for setbacks. Remember, these aren't really failures, they are opportunities for growth! Adjust your plan of attack and workout program to better reach your goals.

78. **Be honest with yourself.** If you skip a workout or do the bare minimum one day, acknowledge it. The only way you will ever replace bad habits with better ones is by admitting that they do actually exist and correcting them.

79. **Get inspired to make positive changes in other areas of your life.** Use the increased confidence you get from working out regularly in other parts of your life. Seek out a new job, ask for a raise, or ask someone out on a date.

80. **Keep your chin up!** When doing exercise moves, running or weight lifting, don't drop your head or hunch over — keep your chin up and eyes forward. This opens airways for better breathing and keeps your energy raised and focused.

81. **Don't let your social life derail your progress.** Too often people skip out on exercise for a social engagement. Of course you'd rather see a movie, get a drink with a friend, or go to a party than work out, but you have to make exercise a priority. Tell friends you'll take a raincheck.

82. **Improve your asthma with regular exercise.** Many people with asthma fear that exercise is not an option for them. However, according to the American Council of Exercise, treadmill running, cycling, walking, and pool swimming are safe and healthy for asthmatics. Check with your doctor, as well.

83. **Try doing cardio during a sporting event or hour-long TV show.** A great way to pass time quickly during a cardio session is by watching a sporting event or hour-long TV show. The time will fly by!

84. **Know that walking is an effective way to incorporate daily exercise.** Both low- and high-intensity exercises have equal potential for burning calories and helping you lose weight. When you don't have energy for a serious gym session, take a brisk walk around your neighborhood for 30 minutes.

85. **Decrease the stress of your everyday life with exercise.** Stress leads to sleeplessness, anxiety, overeating and weight gain. However, fitness is the number one stress reliever, so enjoy the relaxing benefits of a great workout.

86. **Get plenty of sleep.** Sleep helps facilitate muscle growth and strength. Without proper sleep you cannot reach your optimum fitness levels, so for your health and fitness, enjoy 7 to 9 hours a night.

87. **Surround yourself with individuals who share your fitness goals.** Avoid slipping back into a sedentary lifestyle by surrounding yourself with people who share fitness goals similar to yours.

88. **Don't be afraid to push yourself to burn extra calories.** Losing those few extra pounds is often just a matter of pushing yourself for a few extra minutes or a few more reps!

89. **Target belly fat with diet to let ab muscles show through.** Doing endless crunches won't give you 6-pack abs, but losing belly fat by eating a high-fiber, low-fat diet will let your core work show through.

90. **Maintain the intensity of your workouts until you reach your goal weight.** Maintaining your ideal weight will be easier than the hard work it takes to get there. So fight through the 2 weeks of tough workout sessions, knowing you can ease up a bit once you've lost the weight.

91. **Use caffeine 45 minutes before a workout for a jumpstart.** If you need a boost for your workout, try having about 100 mg of caffeine 45 minutes beforehand. Be sure to drink water as well, as caffeine can dehydrate you.

92. **Mix up your music playlist every month.** Your music playlists need a periodic revamp, just like your exercise routine. Download new songs every month to fuel your workouts.

93. **Find a friend who wants to try out a new sport or activity with you.** Thinking about trying a new sport or activity can be scary, but if you find a friend who wants to join you, you'll be more inclined to do it and stick with it.

94. **Don't let alcohol interfere with your success.** There is really no place for alcohol in a 2-week diet and fitness program. Skip the calories and sluggish effect alcohol will have on your body

and hit the gym instead.

95. **Measure your improvement.** Test yourself at the beginning of your program to see how many situps, pushups and squats you can do. Then, test yourself again after 2 weeks and marvel at your improvement. It will be very motivating.

96. **Document progress with pictures.** Take a series of photos throughout your weight-loss journey to visually assess your progress. Wear a one-piece swimsuit to reveal slimmer hips, thighs and waist.

97. **Revisit exercises you have avoided in the past.** You may think you hate running or swimming — maybe because they were difficult for you as a teenager in gym class. However, give those activities another try. You may find you actually enjoy them now that you're a bit older. Never completely rule out any activity.

98. **Try interval training to burn maximum calories.** Interval training sessions, which combine bursts of high intensity and short periods of rest, tap into fat stores and burn more calories and fat in less time than working out at a consistent pace.

99. **Don't rely solely on the scale.** The scale may not paint an accurate picture of your weight because of water retention and muscle gain. Instead of obsessing over the number on the scale, consider your energy level, mood, focus, and newfound feelings of strength.

100. **Focus on the post-workout glow.** Exercise releases endorphins that give you a natural high, help you sleep great, and make your skin glow. To get through a tough workout, concentrate on how amazing you'll feel afterwards.

When the grass looks greener on the other side of the fence, it may be that they take better care of it there.

~ Unknown

Chapter 18

Make the Right Meal

Never think of eating healthier as depriving yourself of your favorite foods! You can still enjoy delicious, filling meals, such as pizza, pasta, pancakes, and much more by using the ingredient substitutions in this chapter. Take a look at the high calorie count of the original recipe, opt for the *Lose Up To 10 Pounds in 2 Weeks* version instead, and you'll save hundreds of calories while still getting the flavors you love. And each meal and snack comes with an even leaner option if you want to cut back even more.

You'll never have to cross burgers, tacos, happy hour, or even fish and chips off your meal plan or wonder what to serve your family for dinner! Just eat smarter, in smaller portions, and build your own healthy versions of the snacks, sides and entrées you crave.

Backyard BBQ Burger

Grilling a juicy burger with all the fixings can make your mouth water just thinking about it, although you won't be doing your waistline any favors. However, you don't have to skip the backyard barbecue — a 4-ounce patty with a few substitutions means you can enjoy a delicious burger meal without all the calories.

Save 374 Calories!

GOOD CHOICE

Lean turkey patty	150
Low-fat Jack cheese	60
Diced green chiles	5
Avocado slices	50
Lettuce, tomato & red onion	10
Southwest spicy mustard	10
Sandwich thin	100
Sweet potato fries	150
TOTAL	**535**

BAD CHOICE

Beef patty	251
Cheddar cheese	113
Bacon, 2 slices	80
Mayonnaise	90
Lettuce, tomato & red onion	10
Ketchup	15
Bun	120
French fries	230
TOTAL	**909**

Go even leaner!

Substitute a portobello mushroom cap (just 36 calories!) for the burger patty and serve a small salad (50 calories) in place of fries.

Asian Chicken Salad

Sugary dressings, calorie-packed toppings and breaded chicken can turn an Asian Chicken Salad into salad sabotage. Swap in grilled chicken, substitute fresh produce for crunchy, fried toppings, and opt for light dressing and you'll have a complete lunch or dinner that's healthy, fresh and filling. You can enjoy even the more calorie-dense toppings, such as edamame and almonds, because they're full of fiber, healthy fats, and protein.

Save 675 Calories!

GOOD CHOICE

Field greens	30
Grilled chicken strips	140
Cabbage	22
Mandarin oranges	80
Edamame	35
Cilantro	10
Slivered almonds, ½ portion	80
Sesame seeds	13
Salad Spritzers Asian Vinaigrette	10
TOTAL	**420**

BAD CHOICE

Field greens	30
Breaded chicken strips	295
Wonton strips	140
Rice noodles	130
Slivered almonds	160
Peanut sauce	160
Asian sesame vinaigrette	180
TOTAL	**1,095**

Go even leaner!

If you can live without a few of the additions to the healthy version of this salad, you can save an additional 100 calories or more.

Tacos Deliciosos

Tacos are a favorite food of many people because they're fast and easy and the options are endless. Choose the best tortilla (soft corn tortillas instead of crunchy taco shells), and the right fillings and toppings and you'll have a low-calorie, low-fat meal that is healthy and tastes amazing.

Save 282 Calories!

GOOD CHOICE

Ground beef-style

soy crumbles	100
Corn tortillas, 2	140
Avocado slices	50
Lettuce & tomato	7
Salsa	8
Black beans	100

TOTAL 405

BAD CHOICE

Ground beef	240
Hard taco shells, 2	260
Shredded Mexican-style cheese	120
Sour cream	60
Lettuce & tomato	7

TOTAL 687

Go even leaner!

To save another 100 calories, use the black beans as your protein filling instead of as a side. Black bean and avocado tacos are vegetarian, low-fat, fiber-filled, and delicious!

Healthy Holiday Meal

Holidays are notorious diet-sabotagers because of the high-calorie, creamy, fatty or sweet dishes. In addition, time with family and friends usually means physical activity is at a low point. You can thoroughly enjoy your next Thanksgiving or holiday get-together without guilt by choosing half portions of some foods, filling up on healthier sides, and either passing on or choosing very small portions of high-calorie items. Note that holidays are the few times a year that your calorie total for one meal should be this high.

Save 1,279 Calories!

GOOD CHOICE

Turkey, no skin, 3 oz. . . . 120
Defatted gravy 100
Stuffing, ½ portion 85
Mashed potatoes 170
Green beans 44
Pumpkin pie 315
Fat-free whipped
topping 15

TOTAL 849

BAD CHOICE

Turkey with skin, 6 oz. . . 320
Gravy 188
Stuffing 170
Sweet potato
casserole 460
Green bean casserole . . 190
Buttered crescent roll . . . 180
Cranberry sauce 110
Pecan pie 510

TOTAL 2,128

Go even leaner!

Fill up on veggies instead of high-carb potatoes. Skip the pie all together and opt for a small bowl of fresh fruit with whipped topping to save 300 calories easily.

Pasta Perfection

Pasta becomes a diet dealbreaker from huge portions, unhealthy topping, and sugary or creamy sauces. Make up for a smaller amount of actual pasta with lean proteins, lots of vegetables, and a garlicky or spicy sauce. Also, stick with whole-grain pastas, which provide dietary fiber and important nutrients not found in regular pasta noodles. Make your own slice of garlic bread and avoid the freezeraisle versions, which are full of oil, salt, and butter.

Save 370 Calories!

GOOD CHOICE

Whole wheat rotini	200
Baked chicken	145
Tomato & garlic sauce	50
Skim-milk ricotta	70
Baby spinach	35
Toasted bread rubbed with fresh garlic clove	80
TOTAL	**580**

BAD CHOICE

Regular rotini	200
Italian sausage	290
Vodka cream sauce	150
Shredded mozzarella	120
Garlic-cheese bread	190
TOTAL	**950**

Go even leaner!

Substitute shredded Parmesan cheese for the thicker ricotta — one tablespoon has only about 20 calories. A small side salad in place of garlic bread can save even more calories, if you're still looking to cut back.

Brown Bag Turkey Sandwich Lunch

Making a lunch instead of eating out can save you hundreds of calories, but only if you put together a healthy sandwich and sides that won't add unnecessary calories to your day. A variety of healthy items will help you feel happy and satiated and won't put you in a mid-afternoon slump.

Save 613 Calories!

GOOD CHOICE

Whole wheat pita	140
Turkey	90
Hummus	40
Lettuce & tomato	7
Light popcorn	30
Nonfat flavored yogurt	120
TOTAL	**427**

BAD CHOICE

Deli bagel	370
Turkey	90
Swiss cheese, 2 slices	220
Mayonnaise	90
Potato chips	150
Chocolate chip cookie	120
TOTAL	**1,040**

Go even leaner!

Want to skip the bread portion of this lunch? Leave out the pita and use the rest of the sandwich ingredients to make a roll-up inside deli slices of turkey. Add a little mustard (just 5 calories) for dipping.

Sweet Treat

Everyone needs a little sweetness sometimes, and as long as you choose the right dessert, you can still stay within your calorie budget and save dozens of grams of fat and sugar. If you're planning on having a dessert, leave one item off your main meal and look forward to your sweet treat.

Save 300 Calories!

GOOD CHOICE

Sugar-free chocolate and
vanilla pudding cup 60
Fat-free whipped
topping 15

_____

TOTAL........... 75

BAD CHOICE

Small hot fudge
sundae 330
Chopped peanuts 45

_____

TOTAL........... 375

Go even leaner!

Leave off the whipped topping if you must, but really, any dessert or snack under 100 calories is a winner!

Perfect Party Dip

Whether you're hosting a soiree or bringing a side dish to a friend's get-together, you should always provide or make one healthy dip that will help you stay within your calorie budget. Swapping Greek ingredients (Mediterranean food is some of the freshest and healthiest in the world) in place of traditional 5- or 7-layer Mexican bean dip makes this a party-favorite without all the fat, carbs and calories.

Save 114 Calories!

GOOD CHOICE

Greek yogurt	120
Kalamata olives	45
Feta	70
Red pepper	29
Cucumbers	8
Romaine lettuce	3
Paprika	6

TOTAL 281

BAD CHOICE

Refried beans	100
Shredded Mexican-style cheese	120
Sour cream	60
Guacamole	83
Black olives	25
Lettuce & tomato	7

TOTAL 395

Go even leaner!

Just 1 ounce of tortilla chips is more than 170 calories! Serve the Mediterranean dip with toasted pita triangles instead to save about 100 calories. Just cut a small pita pocket into 4 sections and toast.

All-American Breakfast

It's called "the most important meal of the day" for a reason. A hearty breakfast is crucial to weight loss, but it's easy to overdo it, so skip the high-fat, high-calorie foods and include whole grains, protein, and fruits and vegetables for a balanced meal. Just look how many more food items you can enjoy with the healthy breakfast option below, with hundreds fewer calories!

Save 262 Calories!

GOOD CHOICE

Turkey bacon, 2 slices . . . 70
Egg whites, 2 50
Mushrooms. 15
Artichoke hearts 45
Whole wheat
English muffin 130
I Can't Believe It's
Not Butter spray 0
Sugar-free fruit jelly 10
Banana 105
Lite orange juice 50

TOTAL . . . . (. 475)

BAD CHOICE

Sausage, 2 links 160
Eggs, 2 126
Cheddar cheese 110
Croissant 231
Orange juice 110

TOTAL 737

Go even leaner!

Even the healthier breakfast option is a big meal. Don't need all that food? Save the English muffin and jam or the banana for your mid-morning snack and cut up to 140 calories from this meal instantly.

Southwest Taco Salad

Taco salads are really a salad imposter, since they typically include high-fat and high-calorie toppings, not to mention being served in a tempting fried tortilla shell. Build your own version of this tasty dish, hold the unhealthy extras, watch your portion size, and you'll have a delicious lunch or dinner on your hands. And don't forget that salsa or hot sauce are always super-low-calorie options to substitute for dressings on salads, baked potatoes and more.

Save 580 Calories!

GOOD CHOICE

Chopped romaine lettuce	30
Lean ground turkey	160
Black beans	100
Fat-free sour cream	30
Avocado slices	50
Diced tomatoes	5
Jalapeños	20
Cilantro	10
Taco sauce	5

TOTAL 410

BAD CHOICE

Taco salad shell	200
Chopped romaine lettuce	30
Shredded beef	180
Refried beans	100
Mexican-style rice	200
Shredded Mexican-style cheese	120
Sour cream	60
Catalina dressing	100

TOTAL 990

Go even leaner!

Soy crumbles taste just like meat but will save you 60 calories more from the healthy meal option. Serve yourself a half-portion of black beans for an additional calorie cut.

Cozy Cocoa

Nothing is better than a soothing cup of hot cocoa on a cold day; however, milk, creamy half and half, chocolate, sugar, and extras like whipped cream mean hundreds of calories per mug. Slim down by swapping in sugar-free mix but including cocoa powder and Hershey's chocolate syrup for real chocolate taste. Add about 20 mini marshmallows, and you won't believe that this decadent treat comes in at under 200 calories.

Save 318 Calories!

GOOD CHOICE

Sugar-free hot chocolate mix	25
Powdered creamer	16
Cocoa powder	20
Hershey's chocolate syrup	50
Mini marshmallows	40
TOTAL	**151**

BAD CHOICE

2% milk	137
Half and half	79
Semisweet chocolate, chopped	70
Brown sugar	35
Vanilla	6
Sugar	60
Whipped cream	82
TOTAL	**469**

Go even leaner!

Hershey's makes a sugar-free version of their classic chocolate syrup that contains just 15 calories per serving. Use that and halve or leave off the marshmallows for an even leaner drink.

Fit Fish & Chips

It's no surprise that the English pub classic fish and chips is a deep-fried, calorie-filled glut. But by using a Japanese breadcrumb called panko and baking cod fillets, instead of deep frying them in beer batter and cooking oil, you can save hundreds of calories and grams of fat. Replace fried and creamy, mayo-based sides with a baked potato, tangy cocktail sauce and vinegar-based coleslaw, and you'll have a healthy, tasty dinner treat.

Save 548 Calories!

GOOD CHOICE

Cod fillets, 2	180
Panko breadcrumbs	55
Egg Beaters	15
Cocktail sauce	30
Baked sweet potato	103
I Can't Believe It's Not Butter spray	0
Vinegar coleslaw	72
TOTAL	**455**

BAD CHOICE

Cod fillets, 2	180
Beer batter	113
Eggs	80
Deep fry oil	100
Tartar sauce	140
French fries	230
Creamy coleslaw	160
TOTAL	**1,003**

Go even leaner!

Cut your portion size in half and fill up on an additional vegetable, such as peas (68 calories) or steamed carrots (30 calories).

Pancake-House Breakfast

Everyone loves a hearty pancake-house-style breakfast, but whipped toppings and refined carbs can make your blood sugar skyrocket and then plummet, leaving you hungry a few hours later. Whip up a batch of "Protein Pancakes," which use high-protein ingredients such as wheat flour, sliced almonds, oats, and soy milk to give your body slow-burning energy to last all morning. Real fruit provides good carbs and fiber in place of sugary toppings.

Save 270 Calories!

GOOD CHOICE

Protein Pancakes, 3 275
Sliced banana. 134
Cinnamon 6
Low-sugar syrup. 30
Green tea 0

TOTAL. 445

BAD CHOICE

Waffles, 3 309
Strawberry topping. 100
Whipped cream 82
Maple syrup 104
Coffee with cream
and sugar 120

TOTAL. 715

Go even leaner!

Enjoy 2 pancakes instead of 3 to save more than 90 calories. Or, choose vitamin C- and fiber-packed blueberries instead of a banana. A whole cup of blueberries has just 70 calories, and they can be bought fresh or frozen.

Chili Chowdown

A comfort food or cold-weather favorite, chili can be made dozens of different ways. Choosing the right vegetables, proteins, and sides can save you hundreds of calories while you enjoy a hearty, delicious meal. For instance, serve lean beef chili over a plain baked potato, instead of sirloin chili and cornbread, and you'll cut out more than 200 calories.

Save 215 Calories!

GOOD CHOICE

Lean ground beef	164
Red and green bell peppers	46
Black beans	100
Stewed tomatoes and onions	66
Hot sauce	0
Baked potato, small	128
TOTAL	**504**

BAD CHOICE

Sirloin	210
Black beans	100
Stewed tomatoes and onions	66
Sour cream	60
Shredded cheddar cheese	110
Corn bread	173
TOTAL	**719**

Go even leaner!

Go vegetarian by substituting a few more varieties of beans — kidney, garbanzo, etc. — and several vegetables — carrots, mushrooms, eggplant, etc. — for ground beef and you'll have an even heartier, lower-calorie meal.

Monte Cristo Sandwich

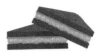

A traditional Monte Cristo sandwich is deep-fried and served with jam, syrup, powdered sugar and more! You can still enjoy this gooey delight without the guilt by grilling the sandwich bread in Egg Beaters and milk, using one slice of flavorful Gruyere instead of two slices of Swiss cheese, and, going easy on the deli meat and sugary toppings. It's a tasty splurge that will keep you in line with your eating plan.

Save 439 Calories!

GOOD CHOICE

Sliced Italian bread	154
Honey ham	120
Gruyere	120
Egg Beaters	15
Skim milk	6
Dijon mustard	10
Sugar-free preserves	10
TOTAL	**435**

BAD CHOICE

French toast	280
Turkey	90
Honey ham	120
Swiss cheese	160
Berry preserves	90
Maple syrup	104
Powdered sugar	30
TOTAL	**874**

Go even leaner!

Cut back to one slice of reduced-fat Swiss cheese (70 calories), or eat only half of the healthy Monte Cristo with a side of fresh fruit or low-fat cottage cheese.

Meatball Sub-stitution

An Italian-deli favorite, the meatball sub is a saucy, cheesy, tasty sandwich that can also wreak havoc on your calorie and fat intake. Subbing in lean turkey meatballs and a whole wheat pita won't detract from the flavor, but will eliminate a lot of the calories. Add mushrooms (or peppers, olives, or any other veggie) to bulk up the fiber.

Save 282 Calories!

GOOD CHOICE

Italian-style turkey
meatballs, 4 160
Shredded parmesan. 20
Sliced mushrooms 8
Red pepper flakes 0
Spicy tomato sauce 60
Whole wheat pita 140

TOTAL. 388

BAD CHOICE

Beef meatballs, 4 210
Provolone cheese,
2 slices 140
Hoagie roll. 220
Marinara sauce. 100

TOTAL. 670

Go even leaner!

Split the pita pocket and eat only half to save 70 calories. You can also cut down to 2 or 3 meatballs and save 40 calories per meatball. In that case, add a small side salad to make a meal complete enough to fill you up.

Eatsa Pizza Pie

No meal plan would be complete without one of the world's favorite foods — pizza! Pass on delivery or frozen pizzas and make your own healthy personal-size pizzas at home. Add as many veggie toppings as you like, just stick to a few low-fat, low-calorie basics, such as light string cheese sticks and a whole wheat pita as your crust (broil it for crispness!).

Save 370 Calories!

GOOD CHOICE

Whole wheat pita	120
Pizza sauce	28
Light string cheese, mozzarella, shredded	50
Turkey pepperoni	36
Black olives	25
Sundried tomatoes	20
Parmesan	20
TOTAL	**299**

BAD CHOICE

Whole wheat pizza crust, 1/3 of pie	250
Pizza sauce	28
Shredded mozzarella	80
Pepperoni	140
Italian sausage	171
TOTAL	**669**

Go even leaner!

As far as pizza goes, it doesn't get much leaner than this — but, replace half a pizza with a light salad with a 10-calorie Spritzer dressing and you've saved 50 calories or more. Enjoy with a Coke Zero or Sprite Zero and you have a low-calorie delicacy!

Better Beef & Broccoli Stir-Fry

Order this classic Asian dish at any restaurant and you're looking at hundreds of calories from oils, sauces, large meat and rice portions, crispy toppings, and more. However, making stir-fry at home, where you can adjust cooking methods, ingredients and portion sizes, makes for a very healthy meal. Just be sure to go easy on the beef and double up on the vegetables to keep the calorie and fat down.

Save 419 Calories!

GOOD CHOICE

Flank steak, 3 oz.	130
Peanut oil	60
Rice, ½ cup.	100
Broccoli, 2 cups	60
Carrots	30
Bean sprouts	15
Sesame oil	40
Chili sauce	20
TOTAL	**455**

BAD CHOICE

Beef, 8 oz.	320
Canola oil	124
Broccoli.	30
Rice, ½ takeout container.	200
Crispy noodles	120
Hoisin sauce.	80
TOTAL	**874**

Go even leaner!

Swap out flank steak for extra-firm tofu and you'll save 50 calories and even more saturated fat. Be sure to go light on the cooking oil you use (use water when you can), and use just a drizzle of sesame oil.

Happy Hour Swap

You don't have to miss out on happy hour celebrations with friends or coworkers just because bar food is typically very unhealthy, in addition to the empty calories in alcohol. Stick to one drink and savor each sip; keeping alcohol to a minimum means that you'll have ingested fewer liquid calories, and the alcohol won't affect your willpower.

Save 530 Calories!

GOOD CHOICE

Light beer 100
Veggies 30
Hummus dip 100

TOTAL 230

BAD CHOICE

Frozen margarita 400
Chips & salsa 360

TOTAL 760

Go even leaner!

Have seltzer water with a squeeze of lemon or lime instead of an alcoholic drink. You'll save calories and won't risk eating more than you need to as the alcohol lowers your inhibitions.

Mid-Afternoon Snack Attack

At a glance, it might not seem like saving 45 calories is much, but the unhealthy snack option below contains simple sugars, refined carbs, and few nutrients, meaning you'll be hungry again soon after eating. Don't be fooled by trail mix and the word "fruit," which lead you to believe you're eating smart! An afternoon snack should give you energy to finish out your day, go for a workout, and fill you up until dinner. Protein, healthy fats, and fiber from natural peanut butter, a medium apple, and light cheese will do the trick, as opposed to hundreds of calories from candy-filled trail mix and sugary fruit snacks.

Save 45 Calories!

GOOD CHOICE

Natural peanut butter . . . 190
Apple 80
Light string cheese 50

TOTAL 320

BAD CHOICE

M&M and peanut
trail mix 280
Fruit snacks 85

TOTAL 365

Go even leaner!

Choose a smaller apple — about ¼ of a pound — and you'll be eating about 55 calories instead of 80.

Big Fat Greek Tuna Sandwich

Tuna may sound like an easy and healthy lunch option, but mayo-packed tuna served on high-calorie sub rolls with cheese (and more mayo!) are some of the least healthy menu items at many restaurants and sandwich shops. Instead, make 5 ounces of tuna Mediterranean-style, serve the sandwich open-faced on one slice of toasted bread, load up on veggies, and enjoy!

Save 205 Calories!

GOOD CHOICE

Tuna	166
Olive oil	40
Dijon mustard	10
Lemon juice	3
Capers	2
Black olives	25
Kalamata olives	45
Feta	70
Roma tomato slices	5
Multigrain bread, 1 slice	85
TOTAL	**451**

BAD CHOICE

Tuna	166
Mayonnaise	160
Pepperjack cheese	100
Lettuce	3
Tomato	2
Red onion	5
Sub roll	220
TOTAL	**656**

Go even leaner!

Skip the bread and serve tuna on a bed of crisp lettuce or spooned into a halved avocado. Avocados are an amazing source of healthy fats, potassium, folate, and vitamin E. They are one of nature's super foods and taste delicious with tuna!

Amazing Asian Noodle Soup

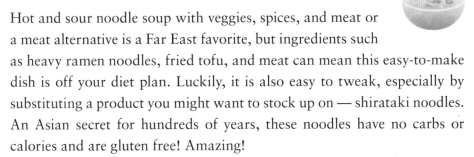

Hot and sour noodle soup with veggies, spices, and meat or a meat alternative is a Far East favorite, but ingredients such as heavy ramen noodles, fried tofu, and meat can mean this easy-to-make dish is off your diet plan. Luckily, it is also easy to tweak, especially by substituting a product you might want to stock up on — shirataki noodles. An Asian secret for hundreds of years, these noodles have no carbs or calories and are gluten free! Amazing!

Save 371 Calories!

GOOD CHOICE

Low-sodium chicken broth	15
Shirataki noodles	0
Lean pork loin, ½ portion	65
Mushrooms	8
Firm tofu	55
White vinegar	0
Low-sodium soy sauce	10
Ground red pepper	0
TOTAL	**153**

BAD CHOICE

Chicken broth	15
Ramen noodles	190
Pork	139
Fried tofu	105
Sherry	30
Soy sauce	10
Hoisin sauce	35
TOTAL	**524**

Go even leaner!

Go vegetarian by skipping the meat and stuffing your soup with vegetables you enjoy — try bok choy, snow peas, carrots, broccoli, or cabbage — for even more fiber.

Weightless Waldorf Salad

From the kitchens of New York's Waldorf Astoria Hotel, this classic is served slightly sweet, as a side dish that can double as a salad or dessert. However, it is traditionally made with mayonnaise, sugar, honey, or fruit juice, making it an unhealthy option. Pass on the creamy, sugary, fatty ingredients, and enjoy a lighter version of this popular summertime salad.

Save 288 Calories!

GOOD CHOICE

Golden Delicious apple, ½	30
Raisins	20
Walnuts	64
Red grapes	25
Celery	4
Low-fat vanilla yogurt	20
Lemon juice	3
Splenda	0
Butter lettuce leaves	2
TOTAL	**168**

BAD CHOICE

Apple, large	100
Mayonnaise	90
Plain yogurt	80
Apple juice	90
Walnuts	64
Grapes	25
Celery	4
Lemon juice	3
TOTAL	**456**

Go even leaner!

Small portions are key to cutting calories and losing weight, so serve a smaller portion of this side salad alongside grilled chicken and a fresh summer vegetable.

Mac 'n' Cheese, Please

A comfort-food staple, traditional mac 'n' cheese fattens up with multiple types of cheese, oil, whole milk, and often an entire stick of butter! Slim down with low-fat ricotta and shredded cheese and replace half the macaroni with oven-baked butternut squash, one of nature's superfoods for being low in fat, high in fiber and potassium, and packed with antioxidants to fight heart disease.

Save 415 Calories!

GOOD CHOICE

Elbow macaroni	72
Butternut squash	37
Onion	4
Skim milk	20
Low-fat shredded cheese	42
Skim-milk ricotta	30
Black pepper	0
TOTAL	**205**

BAD CHOICE

Elbow macaroni	144
Unsalted butter	80
Whole milk	100
Shredded cheddar	56
Shredded Monterey Jack	48
Shredded Muenster	52
Vegetable oil	140
TOTAL	**620**

Go even leaner!

The more spices you use, the fewer high-fat ingredients you'll need. Try incorporating nutmeg, cayenne pepper, sea salt, and even cinnamon for calorie-free flavor.

Applesauce & Carob-Chip Cookies

Replacing the butter and oil in this recipe with applesauce (or even a mashed banana) makes cookies that are chewy and healthy. Carob chips and honey are also perfect substitutes for chocolate and sugar because both are naturally sweet. These hearty oatmeal cookies will be a new healthy favorite for kids and parents alike.

Save 126 Calories!

GOOD CHOICE

Whole wheat flour	20
Rolled oats	25
Applesauce	15
Raisins	15
Carob chips	26
Honey	20
Cinnamon & nutmeg	6
TOTAL	**127**

BAD CHOICE

Flour	35
Rolled oats	25
Butter	62
Sugar	35
Oil	39
Vanilla	6
Walnuts	21
Semi-sweet chocolate	30
TOTAL	**253**

Go even leaner!

Try sugar-free carob chips to cut even more calories. Load up on cinnamon (3 tbsp even!) for extra spice and flavor without adding calories.

Savory Seafood Quiche

The key to keeping quiche healthy is to make it crustless and pack it with delicious veggies like caramelized onions and low-fat cheese. Add a lean protein, such as lump crabmeat and you have a hearty, savory quiche that is the prefect meal for breakfast, lunch or dinner!

Save 232 Calories!

GOOD CHOICE

Egg Beaters Whites	48
Lump crabmeat	45
Skim milk	20
Spinach	35
Fat-free gruyere	45
Mushrooms	8
Onion, slivered	4
Sundried tomatoes	20
TOTAL	**225**

BAD CHOICE

Eggs	55
Bacon	76
Heavy cream	82
Spinach	35
Swiss	76
Onion	4
Pie crust	129
TOTAL	**457**

Go even leaner!

Try to avoid imitation crab, or Krab, which will be higher in both sodium and sugar. If you want vegetarian quiche, you can sub extras veggies (red peppers would be tasty, for instance) and save a few calories.

Guilt-Free Quesadilla

A quesadilla is a quick meal — basically just a tortilla or two that can be stuffed with nearly anything! The problem is, restaurant or fast-food versions are heavy on cheese and slim on other ingredients and are always cooked with at least a tablespoon of butter in the pan. Shop for La Tortilla Factory tortillas, which are high in fiber and super-low in carbs and calories!

Save 364 Calories!

GOOD CHOICE

La Tortilla Factory
tortilla, 1 large. 80
Grilled chicken 70
Low-fat shredded
cheese 36
Red & green peppers . . . 12
Light sour cream 30
Tomatillo salsa 10

TOTAL. 238

BAD CHOICE

Tortillas, 2 240
Butter 102
Grilled chicken 70
Shredded Mexican-style
cheese 120
Sour cream. 60
Salsa. 10

TOTAL. 602

Go even leaner!

Hold the sour cream for even fewer calories, although low-fat or non-fat sour cream is a fine addition to your Mexican-food favorites when eaten in small doses.

Stuffed Peppers

Favorite ingredients baked into tender green peppers make for a delicious, unique dinner, but using lean meat and low-fat cheese in place of high-fat sausage and two types of regular cheese makes it very healthy, too. Melt the mozzarella over the top with a hearty tomato sauce and you've got a saucy, cheesy, baked dish that's sure to be a hit.

Save 240 Calories!

GOOD CHOICE

Green peppers	30
Lean ground turkey	50
Stewed tomatoes	29
Onion	4
Long grain rice	66
Garlic, oregano & basil	6
Low-fat mozzarella	50
TOTAL	**235**

BAD CHOICE

Green peppers	30
Italian sausage	73
Breadcrumbs	60
Long grain rice	66
Marinara sauce	100
Garlic	4
Cheddar cheese	57
Mozzarella	85
TOTAL	**475**

Go even leaner!

Smaller peppers can be filled with less of everything — less rice, meat and cheese — for even fewer calories. You can also serve half portions of this dish with a small side salad.

Best BLT

What could be simpler or tastier than the classic BLT sandwich? However, a smear of full-fat mayo and a high-calorie serving of pasta salad on the side add hundreds of unnecessary calories. Go lean with turkey bacon, Dijonnaise, and a quick side salad of sliced avocado doused with a light spray dressing.

Save 287 Calories!

GOOD CHOICE

Wheat bread	130
Turkey bacon, 2 slices	70
Lettuce	3
Tomato	2
Dijonnaise	15
Avocado slices	50
Italian dressing spritzer	10
TOTAL	**280**

BAD CHOICE

Grain bread	200
Bacon, 2 slices	92
Lettuce	3
Tomato	2
Mayonnaise	90
Pasta salad	180
TOTAL	**567**

Go even leaner!

Try two slices of one of the newer "lite" breads by Sara Lee, Orowheat, Nature's Own, or other brands, which have just 40 to 45 calories per slice, instead of as many as 110 calories per slice. Slices are smaller but provide great whole-wheat flavor.

Strawberry Shortcake Swap

Strawberry shortcake is a dessert that kids and adults love — but it's hard to love all the sugar and calories. Start by substituting a light and fluffy dessert shell for a dense biscuit. Calorie-free Splenda and light whipped topping round out this sweet and fruity treat that comes in at under 200 calories.

Save 214 Calories!

GOOD CHOICE

Angel food cake dessert shell	110
Strawberries	53
Splenda	0
Fat-free whipped topping	15
TOTAL	**178**

BAD CHOICE

Bisquick biscuit	212
Strawberries	53
Sugar	45
Whipped cream	82
TOTAL	**392**

Go even leaner!

A whole cup of sliced strawberries has just 53 calories and is low on the glycemic index, but you can cut the amount in half if you want to go even slimmer with this summertime recipe.

“ You have brains in your head. You have feet in your shoes.
You can steer yourself in any direction you choose. ”

~ Dr. Seuss

Chapter 19

Order the Right Meal

At America's Most Popular Restaurants

Many dieters say that eating out is the number one thing that prevents them from losing weight. It's true that finding a healthy option can be extremely difficult at most restaurants and fast-food chains. That's where this section will come in handy! By providing at-a-glance calorie information for the most healthy and least healthy salads, sides, entrées, appetizers, desserts and beverages from 140 of the nation's most popular restaurants, you will quickly be able to decide where to eat and what to order when dining out. You will save thousands of calories by referring to this chapter!

Losing weight and eating better can still include a delicious dinner at a sit-down restaurant or a meal from the drive-thru — you just need to recognize what your healthy and unhealthy options are and make the right choices. Keep this book close by when you are dining out, compare the healthiest and unhealthiest of your favorite restaurant menu items, and you'll be well on your way to dropping 10 pounds!

A&W RESTAURANT . . . . *SAVE 1530 CALORIES !*

GOOD CHOICE

Strawberry Sundae, 189 g	300
Hotdog (plain), 53 g	.310
A&W Diet Rootbeer	0
Total.	**.610**

BAD CHOICE

Vanilla Milkshake, 594 g	900
Orig Bacon Double Chz burger, 297 g . . .	.760
A&W Rootbeer	290
Total	**2140**

AMAZON CAFÉ . . . . *SAVE 324 CALORIES !*

GOOD CHOICE

Skinny Delight Smoothie, 16 oz.	186
Tomato & Three Cheese Soup, 8 oz.	60
Total.	**.246**

BAD CHOICE

Pina Colada Smoothie, 16 oz.	320
Chili Con Carne, 8 oz.	250
Total	**570**

APPLEBEE'S . . . . *SAVE 2890 CALORIES !*

GOOD CHOICE

Seasonal Vegetables, Side	50
Weight Watchers® Italian Chicken & Portobello	
Sandwich w/ fruit	360
Hot Fudge Sundae Shooter.	340
Total.	**.750**

BAD CHOICE

Breadstick	80
Crispy Orange Chicken Bowl	1900
Chocolate Chip Cookie Sundae	1660
Total	**.3640**

ARBY'S. . . . . *SAVE 1395 CALORIES !*

GOOD CHOICE

Diet Blackberry FruiTea, 327 g	5
Chopped Side Salad, 120 g	.70
Roast Chicken Ranch Sandwich, 211 g . . .	340
Total.	**.415**

BAD CHOICE

Chocolate Swirl Shake, 482 g	630
Jalapeño Bites® (5), 110 g	300
Ultimate BLT Sandwich, 295 g	880
Total	**1810**

ORDER THE RIGHT MEAL AT AMERICA'S MOST POPULAR RESTAURANTS

ATLANTA BREAD COMPANY (BREAKFAST) . . . . . *SAVE 745 CALORIES !*

GOOD CHOICE
Espresso, single shot, 2 oz. 5
Low-Carb Cranberry Walnut Bagel, 2 oz. . . . 110
Scrambled eggs, 6 oz. 220
Ham, 2 oz. 60

Total. 395

BAD CHOICE
Hot Chocolate, tall, 16 oz. 450
Sausage, Egg & Cheese on
  Croissant, 7 oz. 690

Total 1140

ATLANTA BREAD COMPANY (LUNCH) . . . . *SAVE 1390 CALORIES !*

GOOD CHOICE
French Onion Soup, 10 oz. 80
Chicken Salad (Scoop), 4 oz. 280
Boston Cream Pound Cake, 2 oz. 200

Total. 560

BAD CHOICE
Chkn & Dumpling Soup, 10 oz. 290
Chicken Pesto Sandwich, 12 oz. 800
Pecan Roll, 6 oz. 860

Total 1950

AU BON PAIN (BREAKFAST). . . . .*SAVE 1415 CALORIES !*

GOOD CHOICE
Caffe Americano, 16 fl.oz. 10
Roasted Potatoes, 1 oz. 35
Apple Croissant, 4 oz. 280

Total. 325

BAD CHOICE
Caramel Blast Smoothie, 16 fl.oz. 540
Muesli, 8 oz. 390
Pecan Roll, 6 oz. 810

Total 1740

AU BON PAIN (LUNCH) . . . . *SAVE 1315 CALORIES !*

GOOD CHOICE
Garden Salad, 7 oz. 70
1/2 Snd Turkey & Swiss on Farm Roll, 6 oz. 320
Chocolate Covered Strawberry, 1 oz. 35

Total. 425

BAD CHOICE
Baked Stuffed Potato, 12 oz. 350
Prosciutto Mozzarella Sandwich, 12 oz. . .810
Chocolate Orange Pecan Scone, 5 oz. . . . 580

Total 1740

AUNTIE ANNE'S . . . . *SAVE 750 CALORIES !*

GOOD CHOICE		BAD CHOICE	
Poland Springs® Bottled Water, 501 ml	0	Strawberry Dutch Shake, 288 g	600
Heated Marinara Sauce, 60 g	20	Caramel Dip, 40 g	130
Jalapeño Pretzel, 124 g	330	Cinnamon Sugar Party Pretzels, 882 g	370
Total	**350**	**Total**	**1100**

BAKER'S DRIVE-THRU . . . . *SAVE 1650 CALORIES !*

GOOD CHOICE		BAD CHOICE	
Side Salad	45	Fiesta Salad	290
Soft Taco w/Shredded Beef	170	Nachos	1575
Total	**215**	**Total**	**1865**

BD'S MONGOLIAN BARBECUE . . . . *SAVE 758 CALORIES !*

GOOD CHOICE		BAD CHOICE	
Tortillas, 1 ea	90	Noodles, 2 oz	210
Shrimp, 3 oz	65	Sausage, 3 oz	273
Rosemary Chkn & Dumpl Soup, 8 oz	80	Tomato Bisque Soup, 8 oz	320
Cheesecake Mini, 1 oz	220	Peanut Butter Cup Mini, 1 oz	410
Total	**455**	**Total**	**1213**

BEN & JERRY'S . . . . *SAVE 2553 CALORIES !*

GOOD CHOICE		BAD CHOICE	
Italiano Specialty Drink, 16 oz	89	Turtle Mocha, 16 oz	522
Garden Mix Cafe Salad w/o egg, 7 oz	63	Mediterranean Bread Salad, 19 oz	973
French Onion Soup, 8 oz	60	Cheese & Bacon Soup, 8 oz	310
Bruschetta Pizzaah, 13 oz	162	Manhattan Club, 16 oz	1122
Total	**374**	**Total**	**2927**

BLIMPIE . . . . *SAVE 1030 CALORIES !*

GOOD CHOICE		BAD CHOICE	
Garden Salad, 184 g	30	Macaroni Salad, side, 145 g	330
Garden Vegetable Soup, 9 oz.	80	Grande Chili with Bean & Beef, 9 oz.	310
Turkey and Cranberry 6", 279 g	350	Ciabatta, Chicken & Pepperoni, 288 g	710
Oatmeal Raisin Cookie, 2 oz.	180	Sugar Cookie, 3 oz.	320
Total	**640**	**Total**	**1670**

BOB EVANS RESTAURANTS (LUNCH) . . . . *SAVE 1668 CALORIES !*

GOOD CHOICE		BAD CHOICE	
Arnold Palmer, 269 g	47	Caramel Mocha, 283 g	268
Itsy Bitsy Trio, Mini Pot Roast		Itsy Bitsy Sandwich Trio, 454 g	1134
Sandwich, 99 g.	243	Cherry Deep Dish Cobbler, 232 g	667
Vanilla Ice Cream, 79 g	111		
Total	**401**	**Total**	**2069**

BOB EVANS RESTAURANTS (DINNER) . . . . *SAVE 1765 CALORIES !*

GOOD CHOICE		BAD CHOICE	
Home Fries, 145 g	164	Loaded Baked Potato, 329 g	395
Dinner salad with oil and vinegar, 85 g.	54	Country Caesar Salad, 473 g	744
Cup of Vegetable Beef Soup, 179 g.	90	Cup of Sausage Chili, 170 g	215
Grilled Chicken Breast, 113 g	165	Slow-Roasted Chicken Pot Pie, 510 g	884
Total	**473**	**Total**	**2238**

BOJANGLES . . . . *SAVE 913 CALORIES !*

GOOD CHOICE		BAD CHOICE	
Green Beans	25	Seasoned Fries	344
Spiced Chicken Leg	122	Spiced Chicken Thigh	310
Biscuit Sandwich (plain)	243	Steak Biscuit Sandwich	649
Total	**390**	**Total**	**1303**

BOSTON MARKET.......................... *SAVE 1960 CALORIES !*

GOOD CHOICE	
Roasted Turkey Salad, 14 oz.	110
Fresh Steamed Vegetables, 5 oz.	60
Roasted Turkey, 113 g	150
Cornbread, 2 oz.	180
Total.	**500**

BAD CHOICE	
Market Chopped Salad, 3 oz.	480
Sweet Potato Casserole, 7 oz.	460
Boston Meatloaf Carver, 449 g	940
Apple Pie (slice), 6 oz.	580
Total	**2460**

BROWN'S CHICKEN & PASTA .... *SAVE 1025 CALORIES !*

GOOD CHOICE	
Cheezy Potatoes, 12 oz.	188
Potato Salad	95
Chicken Breast	284
Total.	**567**

BAD CHOICE	
Spaghetti (in Marinara)	792
Corn Fritters	415
Chicken Wing	385
Total	**1592**

BRUEGGER'S .... *SAVE 1150 CALORIES !*

GOOD CHOICE	
Spinach & Lentil, 8 oz.	110
Garden Veggie Plain Bagel, 12 oz.	360
Marshmallow Chew, 2 oz.	280
Total.	**750**

BAD CHOICE	
Chicken Wild Rice, 8 oz.	280
Tuna & Cheddar Melt / Honey Wheat Panini, 12 oz.	970
Seven Layer Bar, 5 oz.	650
Total	**1900**

BUCA DI BEPPO .... *SAVE 2127 CALORIES !*

GOOD CHOICE	
Espresso, 5 oz.	1
Green Beans	91
Mixed Green Salad	159
Veal Parmigiana	287
Total.	**538**

BAD CHOICE	
Sassy Strawberry Cream Soda, 11 oz.	497
Italian Sausage & Peppers	512
Lunch Soup & Caesar Salad	648
Chicken Carbonara	1008
Total	**2665**

BURGER KING. . . . . *SAVE 810 CALORIES !*

GOOD CHOICE
Hamburger, 110 g 275
BK Fusions® Strawberry Chzcake, 170 g . 345

Total. 620

BAD CHOICE
Double WHOPPER® w/ Chz, 380 g . . . 963
Regular BK® Shake (Chocolate), 401 g 467

Total .1430

BURGERVILLE, USA . . . . *SAVE 1580 CALORIES !*

GOOD CHOICE
Side Salad, 119 g 50
Nine Grain Turkey Club Sandwich
    w/o mayo or cheese, 173 g 300
Triple Berry YoCream Sundae, 170 g 200

Total. 550

BAD CHOICE
Grilled Chicken Salad, 366 g 420
Pepper Bacon Cheeseburger, 259 g . . . 680
Cherry Chocolate Milkshake, 16 g 1030

Total .2130

CAPTAIN D'S SEAFOOD . . . . *SAVE 1817 CALORIES !*

GOOD CHOICE
Broccoli, 100 g 40
Side Salad, 232 g 19
Fish or Chicken Only 10 Pc, 213 g 400

Total. 459

BAD CHOICE
Hush Puppies, 99 g 400
Bite Size Shrimp Salad, 317 g 267
Deluxe Seafood Platter, 606 g 1609

Total .2276

CARL'S JR. . . . . *SAVE 2080 CALORIES !*

GOOD CHOICE
Chicken Stars™ (4 pieces), 56 g 210
Kid's Hamburger, 102 g 230
Strawberry Swirl Cheesecake, 99 g 290

Total. 730

BAD CHOICE
Chili Cheese Fries, 344 g 980
The Guacamole Bacon 6 Dollar
    Burger®, 411 g 1040
OREO® Cookie Malt, 414 g 790

Total .2810

CHARLEY'S GRILLED SUBS. . . . . *SAVE 346 CALORIES !*

GOOD CHOICE
Fresh Garden Salad 58
Philly Veggie Sandwich. 449

Total. .507

BAD CHOICE
Chicken Teriyaki Salad 213
Sicilian Steak Sandwich 640

Total 853

CHEVY'S FRESH MEX. . . . . *SAVE 1915 CALORIES !*

GOOD CHOICE
Original Chicken Fajitas 360
Sopapillas. 550

Total. .910

BAD CHOICE
Grande Chimi Beef Burrito 1725
Deep Fried Ice Cream 1100

Total .2825

CHICK-FIL-A . . . . *SAVE 1100 CALORIES !*

GOOD CHOICE
Side Salad, 113 g 70
Chargrilled Chicken Sandwich, 228 g 300
Icedream Cone, 135 g 170

Total. .540

BAD CHOICE
Cole Slaw, 149 g 290
Chick-n-Strips: 4-count, 218 g 500
Peach Milkshake, 595 g 850

Total .1640

CHILI'S RESTAURANT. . . . . *SAVE 3745 CALORIES !*

GOOD CHOICE
Side Corn Cob w/o Butter 35
Chicken & Green Chili Soup 190
Margarita Grilled Chicken 110
Sweet Shot, Key Lime Pie 240

Total. .575

BAD CHOICE
Loaded Mashed Potatoes 390
Chili's Terlingua Chili w/ Toppings. 460
Jalapeño Smokehouse Burger
   w/ Jalapeño Ranch 2130
Brownie Sundae 1340

Total .4320

CORNER BAKERY CAFÉ (BREAKFAST) . . . . *SAVE 820 CALORIES !*

GOOD CHOICE		BAD CHOICE	
Ham & Swiss Panini w/ Egg Whites	550	Anaheim Breakfast Panini	740
Raisin Pecan Bread	140	Cinnamon Creme Cake, Slice	770
Total	**690**	**Total**	**1510**

CORNER BAKERY CAFÉ (LUNCH) . . . . *SAVE 1730 CALORIES !*

GOOD CHOICE		BAD CHOICE	
Greek Marinated Vegetable Salad	60	Loaded Baked Potato	410
Mom's Turkey on Harvest Bread	410	Pesto Cavatappi	1100
Oatmeal Raisin Cookie	220	Peanut Butter Whoopee Pie	440
Total	**690**	**Total**	**1950**

COSI (BREAKFAST) . . . . *SAVE 1126 CALORIES !*

GOOD CHOICE		BAD CHOICE	
Café Americano, 16 oz.	8	Cosi Sangria, 16 oz.	553
Spinach Florentine Breakfast, 11 oz.	334	Pesto Garden Omelette Croissant, 1 oz.	740
Strawberry Parfait, 12 oz.	331	Chocolate Chip Muffin, 147 g	506
Total	**673**	**Total**	**1799**

COSI (LUNCH) . . . . *SAVE 1570 CALORIES !*

GOOD CHOICE		BAD CHOICE	
Lighter Bombay Chicken Salad, 13oz.	188	Shanghai Chicken Salad, 10 oz.	313
Three Bean Chili, 5 oz.	75	Cheese Flatbread Pizza, 14 oz.	887
Stawberry Parfait, 12 oz.	331	Cinnamon Apple Pie, 14 oz.	964
Total	**594**	**Total**	**2164**

COUNTRY BUFFET . . . . *SAVE 585 CALORIES !*

GOOD CHOICE	
Spring Mix, 45 g	5
Chicken Tortilla Soup, 123 g	40
English Muffins, dry, 26 g	60
Total	**105**

BAD CHOICE	
Seafood Salad, 117 g	310
New England Clam Chowder, 123 g	150
Garlic Cheese Biscuit, 60 g	230
Total	**690**

COUSINS SUBS . . . . *SAVE 932 CALORIES !*

GOOD CHOICE	
Side Salad, 124 g	135
Vegetable Beef Soup, 198 g	70
Garden Veggie Sub, 218 g	266
Total	**471**

BAD CHOICE	
Garden Salad w/ Chkn Breast, 227 g	148
Chicken with Wild Rice Soup, 198 g	219
Italian Special Sub, 343 g	817
Total	**1403**

CULVER'S . . . . *SAVE 3155 CALORIES !*

GOOD CHOICE	
Side Caesar, 3 oz	54
Hearty Vegetable Soup, 227 g	40
Flame-Roasted Chicken Sandwich, 7 oz	308
Lemon Ice, 196 g	84
Total	**486**

BAD CHOICE	
Chicken Cashew Salad, 12 oz	443
Wild & Brown Rice w/ Chkn Soup, 11 oz	452
Steak Bomb Sub, 896 g	1590
Turtle Concrete Mixer, 15 oz	1156
Total	**3641**

DAIRY QUEEN . . . . *SAVE 3150 CALORIES !*

GOOD CHOICE	
Breaded Mushrooms, 114 g	250
Grilled Chicken Wrap, 85 g	200
DQ Fudge Bar - no sugar added, 66 g	50
Total	**500**

BAD CHOICE	
Chili Cheese Fries, 504 g	1240
Chicken Strip Basket™ w/Gravy, 432 g	1360
Turtle Pecan Cluster Blizzard, 425 g	1050
Total	**3650**

DEL TACO . . . . *SAVE 1270 CALORIES !*

GOOD CHOICE		BAD CHOICE	
Caramel Mocha Hot Coffee, 443 g	280	Premium Caramel Mocha Shake, 443g	720
Nachos, 113 g	370	Deluxe Chili Cheese Fries™, 340 g	610
Hamburger, 143 g	360	Triple Del™ Cheeseburger, 342 g	950
Total	**1010**	**Total**	**2280**

DENNY'S . . . . *SAVE 1467 CALORIES !*

GOOD CHOICE		BAD CHOICE	
Straight Up Lemon Tea Chiller, 15 oz.	90	Milkshake, 12 oz.	560
Garden Salad w/o dressing, 7 oz.	113	Country-Fried Potatoes, 5 oz.	390
Grilled Chicken, 10 oz.	280	Country-Fried Steak w/ gravy, 13 oz.	1000
Total	**483**	**Total**	**1950**

DON PABLO'S . . . . *SAVE 2801 CALORIES !*

GOOD CHOICE		BAD CHOICE	
Dip Sampler - Guacamole, 2 oz.	83	Dip Sampler, 4, 2 oz. dips	519
Chicken Relleno	235	Cool Amigo Steak Quesadilla	1622
Fried Ice Cream.	424	Sopapillas.	1402
Total	**742**	**Total**	**3543**

DONATOS PIZZA . . . . *SAVE 2017 CALORIES !*

GOOD CHOICE		BAD CHOICE	
Chicken Strips Appetizer, 2 Strips	125	Spicy Garlic Buffalo Wings, 5 Wings	713
Side Harvest Salad	81	Chicken Harvest Salad	410
Chicken Vegy Medley Pizza, 2 slices	281	Meatball Oven-Baked Sub	1119
Cinnamon Twists, 2 pieces	260	Cinnamon Timpano, 2 slices	523
Total	**747**	**Total**	**2765**

DUNKIN DONUTS (BREAKFAST) . . . . *SAVE 1410 CALORIES !*

GOOD CHOICE		BAD CHOICE	
Hazelnut Coffee, 10 fl.oz. 10		Vanilla Bean Coolatta®, 24 fl.oz. 650	
Egg White & Cheese Wake-Up Wrap 150		Sausage, Egg & Cheese on Croissant . . 640	
Sugar Raised Donut, 1 Donut 190		Blueberry Crumb Donut, 1 Donut 470	
Total. . . . .**.350**		**Total** **1760**	

DUNKIN DONUTS (LUNCH). . . . . *SAVE 710 CALORIES !*

GOOD CHOICE		BAD CHOICE	
Decaffeinated Tea, 10 fl.oz. 0		Sweet Tea, 16 fl.oz. 120	
Garden Salad, 12 oz. 180		Chicken Caesar Salad, 10 oz. 440	
Turkey and Bacon Club Sandwich 440		Tuna Melt Sandwich. 770	
Total. **620**		**Total** **1330**	

EAT N' PARK . . . . *SAVE 2174 CALORIES !*

GOOD CHOICE		BAD CHOICE	
Mixed Vegetables 28		French Fries 352	
Chili 208		Cream of Broccoli Soup 380	
Cod Floridian, 2 fillets 241		Black Angus Superburger 1086	
Sherbet 102		Turtle Sundae 935	
Total. . . . .**.579**		**Total** . . . .**.2753**	

EDO JAPAN . . . . *SAVE 1680 CALORIES !*

GOOD CHOICE		BAD CHOICE	
Tofu, 106 g. 90		Rice Side Dish, 279 g 480	
Vegetable Udon Soup, 909 g 370		Beef Udon Soup, 947 g 580	
Grilled Vegetables Teriyaki, 342 g 380		Beef and Shrimp Teriyaki, 486 g 690	
Total. **840**		**Total** **1750**	

EINSTEIN BROS. BAGELS (BREAKFAST) .... *SAVE 1159 CALORIES !*

GOOD CHOICE		BAD CHOICE	
Cafe Americano, 8 fl.oz.	1	Mocha, Whole Milk, 16 fl.oz.	400
Pumpernickel Bagel, 101 g	240	Bacon & Spinach Panini, 348 g	860
Plain Reduced Fat Cream Cheese, 20 g	60		
Total.	**301**	**Total**	**1460**

EINSTEIN BROS. BAGELS (LUNCH). .... *SAVE 1580 CALORIES !*

GOOD CHOICE		BAD CHOICE	
Harney Tropical Green Tea, 8 fl.oz.	0	Blackberry Lemonade, 16 fl.oz.	310
Chicken Noodle, 248 g	120	Vegetarian Broccoli Cheese, 248 g	290
Veg Out on Sesame Seed Bagel, 268 g.	440	Bros Bistro Salad with Chicken, 397 g	940
Mini Oatmeal Raisin Cookie, 39 g	160	Chocolate Chip Coffee Cake, 174 g	760
Total.	**720**	**Total**	**2300**

EL POLLO LOCO .... *SAVE 1095 CALORIES !*

GOOD CHOICE		BAD CHOICE	
6" Corn Tortillas, 2 each.	120	6.5" Flour Tortillas, 2 each	210
Flame-Grilled Chicken Legs, 2	180	Ultimate Pollo Bowl®, 24 oz.	1050
Caramel Flan, 5 oz.	260	Vanilla Regular Cone	320
Total.	**560**	**Total**	**1660**

FAZOLI'S .... *SAVE 1265 CALORIES !*

GOOD CHOICE		BAD CHOICE	
Broccoli, 3 oz.	25	Meatballs, 3 oz.	250
Ravioli w/ Marinara Sauce, 12 oz.	490	Tortellini Robusto, 18 oz.	1020
Chocolate Chip Cannolis, 1 oz.	190	Chocolate Layer Cake, 7 oz.	700
Total.	**705**	**Total**	**1970**

FIREHOUSE SUBS. . . . . *SAVE 940 CALORIES !*

GOOD CHOICE

Unsweetened Tea	0
Veggie Sub, 4 oz.	300
Oreo cookies, 2	110
Total	**410**

BAD CHOICE

Sweetened Tea	170
Chicken Salad Sub, 4 oz.	760
Brownie, 1	420
Total	**1350**

FUDDRUCKERS. . . . . *SAVE 2527 CALORIES !*

GOOD CHOICE

Fruit Cup	60
Veggie Burger w/ Wheat Bun	395
Ice Cream Cookie Sandwich	70
Total	**525**

BAD CHOICE

Onion Rings	566
Three Cheese Burger w/ Bun, 1/2 lb	1121
Ice Cream Brownie Blast	1365
Total	**3052**

GOLD STAR CHILI . . . . *SAVE 1484 CALORIES !*

GOOD CHOICE

Tex Mex Side, 227 g	210
Caesar Salad, 168 g	130
Chili Sandwich, 132 g	211
Total	**551**

BAD CHOICE

Chili Cheese Fries, 269 g	596
South of the Border Chili Salad, 472 g	639
Crispy Chicken Burrito, 277 g	840
Total	**2035**

GOLDEN CORRAL. . . . . *SAVE 1130 CALORIES !*

GOOD CHOICE

Vegetable Beef Soup, 227 g	80
Macaroni and beef, 120 g	110
Sugar Free Strawberry, Cherry, Raspberry Gelatin, 85 g	10
Total	**200**

BAD CHOICE

Loaded Potato & Bacon Soup, 240 g	250
BBQ Chicken leg, 221 g	490
Gourmet Choco Cake w/Choco Frosting, 147g	590
Total	**1330**

GREAT STEAK & POTATO . . . . *SAVE 1470 CALORIES !*

GOOD CHOICE	
Plain Baked Potato, 170 g	160
Salad, Side, 173 g	30
Chicken Philly Slider, 153 g	300
Total	**490**

BAD CHOICE	
King Fry, 324 g	630
Great Salad, Grilled Steak, 551 g	400
Super Steak Cheesesteak, 448 g	930
Total	**1960**

GREEN BURRITO . . . . *SAVE 1490 CALORIES !*

GOOD CHOICE	
Guacamole, 40 g	60
Cheese Quesadilla, 114 g	370
Chicken Hard Taco, 2	280
Total	**610**

BAD CHOICE	
Chips & Cheese, 142 g	700
Super Nachos - Ground Beef, 472 g	1080
Fish Taco, 178 g	320
Total	**2100**

HARDEE'S . . . . *SAVE 1880 CALORIES !*

GOOD CHOICE	
Side Salad (no dressing), 191 g	120
Hot Ham 'N' Cheese™, 131 g	280
Choco Chip Cookie Fresh Baked, 52 g	250
Total	**650**

BAD CHOICE	
Natural-Cut French Fries, 162 g	430
2/3 LB Monster Thickburger®, 386 g	1320
Hand-Scooped Malt, 414 g	780
Total	**2530**

HEAVENLY HAM . . . . *SAVE 360 CALORIES !*

GOOD CHOICE	
Tomato & Cucumber Salad	60
Glazed Bnlss Smoked Turkey Breast, 3 oz.	60
Oatmeal Raisin Nut Cookie	260
Total	**380**

BAD CHOICE	
Heavenly Seven Bean Soup, 1 cup	150
Whole Roasted Turkey, 3 oz.	160
Fudge Brownie	430
Total	**740**

HOT DOG ON A STICK . . . . *SAVE 1015 CALORIES !*

GOOD CHOICE

Sugar Free Lemonade	15
Turkey Hot Dog on a Stick, 92 g	240
Funnel Cake Sticks, 51 g	220
Total	**475**

BAD CHOICE

Lime Lemonade	250
Beef Hot Dog on a Bun, 134 g	460
Zucchini Platter, 279 g	780
Total	**1490**

ISLANDS . . . . *SAVE 2580 CALORIES !*

GOOD CHOICE

Spinach-Artichoke Dip w/Chips, 4 oz.	290
Grilled Veggie Tacos, 2	600
Ice Cream Sundae, 5 oz.	340
Total	**1230**

BAD CHOICE

Beachside Sliders Appetizer, 20 oz.	1490
Mavericks Burger, 22 oz.	1570
Fudge Brownie, 7 oz.	750
Total	**3810**

JACK IN THE BOX . . . . *SAVE 1130 CALORIES !*

GOOD CHOICE

Iced Coffee, Caramel, 24 oz.	150
Fruit Cup, 116 g	50
Grilled Chicken Strips (4 pc.), 198 g	240
Total	**440**

BAD CHOICE

Smoothie, Tropical, 16 oz.	330
Seasoned Curly Fries	280
Sirloin Cheeseburger w/ Bacon, 374 g	960
Total	**1570**

JIMBOY'S TACOS . . . . *SAVE 1315 CALORIES !*

GOOD CHOICE

Fruit Cup	80
Shredded Beef Taco	190
Cinnamon Churros, 3	330
Total	**600**

BAD CHOICE

Parmesan Mini-Dillas	480
Steak Super Nachos	1030
Creme-Filled Churros, 3	405
Total	**1915**

JOHNNY ROCKETS . . . . *SAVE 2384 CALORIES !*

GOOD CHOICE

Side Salad, 113 g	.100
Hot Dog, 142 g	.370
A la mode, 113 g	250

Total. .270

BAD CHOICE

Garden Salad, 312 g	.240
Bacon Cheddar Double, 510 g	1400
The Perfect Brownie Sundae, 425 g . . .	1464

Total 3104

KENTUCKY FRIED CHICKEN . . . . *SAVE 1075 CALORIES !*

GOOD CHOICE

House Side Salad w/o Dressing, 87 g	.15
KFC Snacker®, Honey BBQ, 98 g	.210
Sweet Life® Oatmeal Raisin Cookie, 35 g . .	.150

Total. .375

BAD CHOICE

Crispy Chkn BLT Salad w/o Drss, 315 g.	340
KFC Famous Bowls®-Mashed Potato	
w/ Gravy, 525 g	700
Pecan Pie Slice, 95 g	.410

Total 1450

KOO KOO ROO . . . . *SAVE 1232 CALORIES !*

GOOD CHOICE

Steamed Vegetables, 4 oz.	38
Tossed Salad w/o dressing, 3 oz.	.16
Sliced Turkey Breast	.182

Total. .236

BAD CHOICE

Macaroni & Cheese, 6 oz.	340
BBQ Chicken Salad	365
Chicken Caesar Sandwich	781

Total 1486

LA ROSA'S PIZZERIA . . . . *SAVE 2007 CALORIES !*

GOOD CHOICE

Minestrone Soup, 336 g	.130
Big 4 Veggie Pizza, 106 g	.198
Fudge Brownie Dessert Mini, 40 g	.150

Total. .478

BAD CHOICE

JoJo's BLT Salad, 257 g	505
Ziti Chicken Alfredo, 596 g	982
Italian Crème Cake, 257 g	998

Total .2485

LONG JOHN SILVER . . . . *SAVE 620 CALORIES !*

GOOD CHOICE

Hushpuppies, 23 g	60
Grilled Tilapia, 116 g	110
Chocolate Cream Pie, 74 g	280

Total 450

BAD CHOICE

Jalapeño Cheddar Bites, 82 g	.240
Ultimate Fish Sandwich®, 206 g	530
Pineapple Cream Pie, 89 g	300

Total .1070

MACARONI GRILL . . . . *SAVE 2700 CALORIES !*

GOOD CHOICE

Caesar Salad	260
Jumbo Shrimp Spiedini	230
Italian Sorbetto w/ Biscotti	220

Total 590

BAD CHOICE

Chicken Caesar Salad	650
Grilled Pork Chops	.1380
N.Y. Chzcake w/ Caramel Fudge Sauce	.1650

Total .3290

MAX & ERMA'S . . . . *SAVE 409 CALORIES !*

GOOD CHOICE

Fruit Salad, 5 oz.	54
Baby Greens Salad	119
Caribbean Chicken: Lunch Portion	536

Total 709

BAD CHOICE

Garlic Breadstick, 1 Breadstick	.150
Hula Bowl	.319
Black Bean Veggie Burger	649

Total 1118

MAZZIO'S PIZZA . . . . *SAVE 698 CALORIES !*

GOOD CHOICE

Boneless Dippin' Chicken App., 10 ct	.122
Veggie Thin Crust Pizza, 105 g	.180
Cinnamon Sticks w/o sauce, 145 g	626

Total 928

BAD CHOICE

Cheese Dippers Appetizer, 128 g	405
Greek Pizza, 142 g	.414
Cinnamon Sticks w/ sauce, 202 g	.807

Total .1626

MCDONALDS. . . . . *SAVE 1160 CALORIES !*

GOOD CHOICE		BAD CHOICE	
Side Salad, 87 g	20	Premium Southwest Salad, 353 g	430
Hamburger, 100 g	250	Angus Bacon & Cheese, 291 g	790
Apple Dippers, 68 g	35	McFlurry® w/M&M'S® Candies, 348g	620
Total	**305**	**Total**	**1465**

MR. GOODCENTS . . . . *SAVE 1420 CALORIES !*

GOOD CHOICE		BAD CHOICE	
Baked Lays Original, 28 g	130	Fritos Corn Chips, 28 g	320
Veggie Sub, 212 g	290	Chkn Alfredo on Mostaccioli, 510 g	1370
Baked Brownie, 65 g	260	Giant Chocolate Chip Cookie, 71 g	420
Total	**680**	**Total**	**2100**

MR. SUBS . . . . *SAVE 641 CALORIES !*

GOOD CHOICE		BAD CHOICE	
Garden Salad, 184 g	35	Grilled Chicken Caesar, 185 g	160
Garden Vegetable, 250 g	60	Hearty Chilli with Beef, 250 g	231
Veggie Sub, 118 g	180	Sausage & Egg Sandwich, 224 g	505
Oatmeal Raisin, 38 g	160	Double Chocolate Chip, 38 g	180
Total	**435**	**Total**	**1076**

NOAH'S BAGELS. . . . . *SAVE 2010 CALORIES !*

GOOD CHOICE		BAD CHOICE	
Cafe Americano, 8 fl.oz.	0	Macchiato, Whole Milk, 12 fl.oz.	290
Fruit Cup, 312g	140	Egg Salad, 142 g	330
Chicken Noodle Soup, 248 g	110	Tortilla Soup, 248 g	300
Ancho Chicken Wedge Wrap, 260 g	350	Rachel Sandwich, 394 g	1030
Babka, Chocolate, 56 g	100	Chocolate Chip Coffee Cake, 174 g	760
Total	**700**	**Total**	**2710**

ORDER THE RIGHT MEAL AT AMERICA'S MOST POPULAR RESTAURANTS

NOTHING BUT NOODLES . . . . *SAVE 1631 CALORIES !*

GOOD CHOICE
Garden Fresh Salad 110
Shrimp Pesto Florentine 308
Strawberry Puree 65
Total. **483**

BAD CHOICE
Greek Salad 409
Kung Pao Chicken 935
New York Cheesecake 770
Total **2114**

O'CHARLEY'S . . . . *SAVE 3230 CALORIES !*

GOOD CHOICE
House Salad w/o Dressing 120
Chicken Tortilla Soup 150
Broccoli 140
Butchers Cut Steak, 5 oz. 260
Key Lime Pie. .610
Total. **1280**

BAD CHOICE
Black & Bleu Caesar Salad 1050
Over-Loaded Potato Soup. 160
Sweet Potato Fries, 5 oz. 470
Baked Penne Italiano 1700
Cinnamon Sugar Donuts. 1130
Total **4510**

OLD SPAGHETTI FACTORY . . . . *SAVE 2460 CALORIES !*

GOOD CHOICE
Shrimp Spinach & Artichoke Dip, 67 g. 150
Spinach and Cheese Ravioli, 314 g 480
Minestrone Soup, 9 oz. 60
Italian Cream Soda, 213 g 140
Total. **830**

BAD CHOICE
Sicilian Garlic Cheese Bread, 114 g 328
Hearty Mizithra & Brown Butter, 638 g. .1750
Clam Chowder Soup, 9 oz. 370
Chocolate Truffle Mousse Cake, 250 g . 850
Total **3290**

OLIVE GARDEN . . . . *SAVE 3740 CALORIES !*

GOOD CHOICE
Wild Berry Bellini 160
Mussels di Napoli Appetizer 180
Minestrone 100
Spaghetti with Tomato Sauce 250
Sundae 180
Total. **870**

BAD CHOICE
Strawberry-Limoncello Martini. 300
Lasagna Fritta Appetizer 1030
Grilled Chicken Caesar 850
Pork Milanese 1510
Zeppoli Dessert 920
Total **4610**

ON THE BORDER MEXICAN GRILL . . . . *SAVE 2920 CALORIES*

GOOD CHOICE		BAD CHOICE	
Black Beans w/ Cheese	130	Baja Blend Veggies, 1 Serving	210
Veggies w/ Portobello Mushroom Fajitas	210	Dos XX® Fish Tacos	2240
Sopapillas w/ Chocolate syrup, 2	540	Sopapillas, 5	1350
Total.	**880**	**Total**	**3800**

ORANGE JULIUS. . . . . *SAVE 1360 CALORIES !*

GOOD CHOICE		BAD CHOICE	
Cranberry Orange Julius ®, 20 oz.	150	Cocoa Latte Swirl, 20 oz.	960
Salted Pretzel, 66g	160	Nachos, 226 g	550
Chicken Fajita Pita, 222 g	380	Triple Cheese Dog, 176 g	540
Total.	**.690**	**Total**	**.2050**

OUTBACK STEAKHOUSE . . . . *SAVE 3903 CALORIES !*

GOOD CHOICE		BAD CHOICE	
Sautéed Mushrooms	134	Lobster Tail	530
Steamed Broccoli	130	Sweet Potato	590
Teriyaki Marinated Sirloin, 9 oz.	418	Baby Back Ribs & Aussie Fries	2367
Carrot Cake	112	Spotted Dog Sundae	1216
Total.	**.794**	**Total**	**4697**

PANDA EXPRESS . . . . *SAVE 760 CALORIES !*

GOOD CHOICE		BAD CHOICE	
Veggie Spring Roll, 2 rolls	160	Chicken Potsticker, 3 pcs	220
Broccoli Beef, 5 oz.	150	Beijing Beef, 6 oz.	850
Fortune Cookie, 8g	32	Fortune Cookie, 8g	32
Total.	**.242**	**Total**	**1102**

PANERA BREAD (BREAKFAST) . . . . *SAVE 1170 CALORIES !*

GOOD CHOICE

Low Fat Mango Smoothie, 16 fl.oz.	230
Plain Bagel, 4 oz.	290
Reduced Fat Veggie Spread, 1 oz.	60
Apple Cherry Pastry Ring, 3 oz.	220
Total	**800**

BAD CHOICE

Caramel Latte, 16 fl.oz.	600
Asiago Cheese Bagel Breakfast Sandwich	
w/ Sausage, 8 oz.	650
Pecan Roll, 6 oz.	720
Total	**1970**

PANERA BREAD (LUNCH) . . . . *SAVE 1320 CALORIES !*

GOOD CHOICE

Fresh Fruit Cup - Small, 5 oz.	60
Low-Fat Chicken Noodle Soup, 12 oz.	110
Smoked Turkey Breast on Country, 12 oz. .	560
Total	**730**

BAD CHOICE

Fuji Apple w/ Chicken Salad, 14 oz.	520
Mac & Cheese Side, 8 oz.	490
Italian Combo on Ciabatta, 18 oz.	1040
Total	**2050**

PAPA GINO'S . . . . *SAVE 1400 CALORIES !*

GOOD CHOICE

Plain Chicken Wings, 172g	480
Garden Salad	180
Ravioli, 383 g	590
Total	**1250**

BAD CHOICE

Cheese Breadsticks, 378g	970
Chicken Bacon Cheddar Salad	530
Sausage & Pepper Sub Panini	1150
Total	**2650**

PEI WEI ASIAN DINER . . . . *SAVE 1360 CALORIES !*

GOOD CHOICE

Rice Noodles	60
Vietnamese Chicken Salad Rolls	130
Lemon Pepper Shrimp	210
Total	**400**

BAD CHOICE

Fried Rice	410
Pei Wei Spicy Salad	560
Beef Pad Thai	790
Total	**1760**

PETER PIPER PIZZA . . . . *SAVE 456 CALORIES !*

GOOD CHOICE
Wings 110
Side Salad 20
California Veggie Pizza 200

Total. **330**

BAD CHOICE
Garlic Cheese Bread 310
Family Salad, 1 serv. 96
New York 3 Chz w/ Pepperoni. 380

Total 786

PETROS . . . . *SAVE 767 CALORIES !*

GOOD CHOICE
Chicken Chili. 275
Garden Salad, Small 43
Plain Hotdog. 266

Total. **584**

BAD CHOICE
Veggie Chili. 385
Garden Salad, Large 86
Loaded Tostitos™ Ultimate Nachos. 880

Total 1351

PICCADILLY . . . . *SAVE 1715 CALORIES !*

GOOD CHOICE
Cucumber & Tomato Salad. 40
Cauliflower 89
Mesquite Smoked Chicken. 212
Blueberry Pie 314

Total. **655**

BAD CHOICE
Coleslaw. 163
Fried Okra. .242
Beef Ribeye 1353
Chocolate Almond Pie 612

Total 2370

PIZZA HUT. . . . . *SAVE 1770 CALORIES !*

GOOD CHOICE
Traditional All-American Wings 80
Tomato, Mushroom & Jalapeño Fit 'N'
 Delicious Pizza 150
Cinnamon Sticks, no icing 170

Total. **400**

BAD CHOICE
Fried Cheese Sticks 380
Meat Lover's® Personal Pan 1470
Hershey's® Choco Dunkers® w/sauce 320

Total 2170

PIZZA PIZZA . . . . *SAVE 1820 CALORIES !*

GOOD CHOICE		BAD CHOICE	
Boneless Chicken Bites	200	Crispy Breaded Wings	740
Garden Salad	50	Mediterranean Greek Salad.	170
Pesto Amore Pizza	170	Bacon Chicken Mushroom Melt Pizza . .	850
Two-Bite Brownies.	85	Apple Pie Turnover.	220
Total.	**520**	**Total**	**2340**

POLLO TROPICAL . . . . *SAVE 1670 CALORIES !*

GOOD CHOICE		BAD CHOICE	
Caesar Salad, 3 oz.	140	Caribbean Cobb Chicken Salad, 22 oz. .	950
Balsamic Tomatoes, 5 oz.	110	Coleslaw, 8 oz.	570
Churrasco Steak, 4 oz.	170	Roast Pork, 6 oz.	400
Flan, 4 oz.	210	Tres Leches, 5 oz.	380
Total.	**630**	**Total**	**2300**

POPEYE'S CHICKEN & BISCUITS . . . . *SAVE 960 CALORIES !*

GOOD CHOICE		BAD CHOICE	
Green Beans, 100 g	70	Red Beans & Rice, 174 g	320
Mashed Potatoes, no gravy, 113 g	100	French Fries, 88 g	310
Mild Chicken Strips, 94 g	130	Deluxe Spicy Sandwich, 265 g	630
Total.	**300**	**Total**	**1260**

PORT OF SUBS . . . . *SAVE 1272 CALORIES !*

GOOD CHOICE		BAD CHOICE	
Garden Salad, 8 oz.	93	Grilled Chicken Caesar Salad, 13 oz. . . .	541
Vegetarian Sub, no cheese, 7 oz.	238	BBQ Pork Griller, 299 g	782
Brownies, 5 oz.	300	White Chunk Macadamia Nut Cookie, 5 oz.	580
Total.	**631**	**Total**	**1903**

PRET A MANGER . . . . *SAVE 1222 CALORIES !*

GOOD CHOICE		BAD CHOICE	
Corn Chowder, 12 oz.	38	New England Clam Chowder, 12 oz.	.525
Slim Sandwich, Bacon & Avocado	.275	Swedish Meatball Ragu Hot Wrap, 334 g	700
Nuts & Bolts Cookie	.160	Chocolate Cake	.470
Total	**.473**	**Total**	**1695**

QDOBA MEXICAN GRILL . . . . *SAVE 1105 CALORIES !*

GOOD CHOICE		BAD CHOICE	
Grilled Vegetables Taco Salad, 7 oz.	.75	Ground Beef Taco Salad, 7 oz.	255
Tortilla Soup, 8 oz.	90	Grilled Chicken Soup, 9 oz.	.150
Fajita Ranchera Burrito, 6 oz.	205	Beef 3-Cheese Nachos, 13 oz.	1070
Total	**.370**	**Total**	**1475**

QUIZNO'S SUB . . . . *SAVE 900 CALORIES !*

GOOD CHOICE		BAD CHOICE	
Pan Asian Regular Chopped Salad	.170	Rspbry Chipotle Chkn Chopped Salad	.310
Chicken Noodle Soup	60	Chili	.140
Veggie Sammie	.190	Tuna Melt	.870
Total	**.420**	**Total**	**1320**

RANCH 1 . . . . *SAVE 920 CALORIES !*

GOOD CHOICE		BAD CHOICE	
Rice, 4 oz.	.97	Roll, 6 oz.	.175
Steamed Vegetables, 3 oz.	.27	Mandarin Chicken Salad, 19 oz.	.817
Chicken Platter w/ Rice, 11 oz.	.273	Popcorn Chicken, 6 oz.	.325
Total	**.397**	**Total**	**1317**

RED LOBSTER................................ SAVE 3290 CALORIES !

GOOD CHOICE		BAD CHOICE	
Red Rockin' Shirley Temple	170	Alotta Colada	700
Maine Lobster Tail Side	60	Creamy Lobster Baked Potato	370
Manhattan Clam Chowder	80	New England Clam Chowder	230
Shrimp Lover's Scampi	130	Wood-Grilled Salmon BLT, w/ Chips	1110
Warm Chocolate Chip Lava Cookie	170	Chocolate Wave	1490
Total	**610**	**Total**	**3900**

RED ROBIN................................. SAVE 2740 CALORIES !

GOOD CHOICE		BAD CHOICE	
Freckled Lemonade Light, 356 g	68	Peachberry Fruit Cooler, 284 g	260
House Salad, 117 g	38	Side Caesar Salad, 186 g	313
Simply Grilled Chicken Sandwich, 279 g	420	Buffalo Clucks & Fries, 579 g	1696
Birthday Sundae, 146 g	376	Mountain High Mudd Pie, 453 g	1373
Total	**902**	**Total**	**3642**

ROCKFISH SEAFOOD GRILL................... SAVE 990 CALORIES !

GOOD CHOICE		BAD CHOICE	
Shrimp Cocktail	178	Maryland Crab Cakes	522
Mixed Veggies	17	New Potatoes	152
Small Southwest Caesar Salad	251	Roaring River Salmon Salad	462
Chicken	188	U.S. Farm-Raised Catfish	488
Total	**634**	**Total**	**1624**

ROLY POLY.................................. SAVE 943 CALORIES !

GOOD CHOICE		BAD CHOICE	
Just Veggies Salad	95	Frisco Chicken Salad	527
Harvest Melt on Wheat	190	Cherry Pecan Chicken Club	591
Garden Vegetable Soup, 6 oz.	60	Spring Asparagus Soup, 6 oz.	130
Oatmeal Raisin Cookie, 3 oz.	350	White Choco Mac.Nut Cookie, 3 oz.	390
Total	**695**	**Total**	**1638**

ROUND TABLE PIZZA . . . . *SAVE 720 CALORIES !*

GOOD CHOICE		BAD CHOICE	
Honey BBQ Wings, 1 wing	80	Garlic Bread with Cheese, 1 roll	540
Veggie Sandwich, 1 oz.	530	Chicken Club, 1 oz.	700
Guinevere's Garden Delight, 8	200	Montague's All Meat Marvel, 8	290
Total	**810**	**Total**	**1530**

RUBIO'S . . . . *SAVE 1450 CALORIES !*

GOOD CHOICE		BAD CHOICE	
Black Beans, regular, 116 g	100	Guacamole & Chips, 266 g	790
HealthMex Chicken Taco, 141 g	130	Fish Taco Especial, 177 g	320
Chicken Surfside Citrus Salad, 377 g	250	Blackened Mahi Mahi Surfside Citrus Wrapsalada, 453 g	820
Total	**480**	**Total**	**1930**

RUBY TUESDAY . . . . *SAVE 3464 CALORIES !*

GOOD CHOICE		BAD CHOICE	
Berry Fusion	148	Ruby's Root Beer Float	399
Jumbo Lump Crab Cake	68	Dip Trio	467
Avocado Shrimp Salad	610	Carolina Chicken Salad	1151
Barbecue Grilled Chicken	310	Chicken Piccata	1673
Chocolate Chip Cookie - Mini	80	Italian Cream Cake	990
Total	**1216**	**Total**	**4680**

RUNZA . . . . *SAVE 1090 CALORIES !*

GOOD CHOICE		BAD CHOICE	
Iced Tea, 638 g	0	Smoothie - Banana	220
Vegetable Beef Soup, 270 g	110	Wisconsin Cheese Soup, 299 g	430
Side Salad, 129 g	30	Tossed Salad with Crispy Chkn, 360 g	440
Deluxe Chkn Snd - Grilled, 207 g	380	BBQ Chkn Snd - Crispy, 196 g	520
Total	**520**	**Total**	**1610**

SAMURAI SAM'S TERIYAKI GRILL. . . . . *SAVE 1500 CALORIES !*

GOOD CHOICE	
Grilled Chkn & Veg Eggroll, 85 g.	.140
Veggies, 71 g.	20
Side Salad, 71 g.	.10
Veggie, Brown Rice Bowl, 369 g.	320
Total.	**490**

BAD CHOICE	
California Roll, 170 g	260
Yakisoba Noodles, 227 g	.370
orietnal Chicken Salad, 326 g	340
Sumo Bowl, Brown Rice Bowl, 808 g . .1020
Total	**1990**

SCHLOTZSKY'S. . . . . *SAVE 1535 CALORIES !*

GOOD CHOICE	
Original Baked Crisps.	.140
Side Salad	26
Hearty Vegetable Beef Soup.	60
Fresh Veggie Sandwich	484
Oatmeal Raisin Cookie.	.150
Total.	**860**

BAD CHOICE	
Barbeque Chips.	220
Turkey Chef.	309
Boston Clam Chowder	.175
Albuquerque Turkey Sandwich	.974
Carrot Cake.	.717
Total	.**2395**

SHEETZ . . . . *SAVE 1316 CALORIES !*

GOOD CHOICE	
Fat Free French Vanilla Cupo'ccino, 12 g . . .105
Jalapeño Poppers, 103 g.	.310
Garden Salad, 154 g	.27
Turkey Sandwich, 102 g.	164
Chocolate No Bakes	180
Total.	.**786**

BAD CHOICE	
Shmart Frozen Mocha, 16 g	366
Appetizer Sampler, 192 g.	508
Grilled Chicken Caesar Salad, 145 g . . .	365
Chicken Salad Sandwich, 143 g	363
Old Fashion Chocolate Cake	530
Total	.**2132**

ORDER THE RIGHT MEAL

AT AMERICA'S MOST POPULAR RESTAURANTS

SHONEY'S . . . . *SAVE 1678 CALORIES !*

GOOD CHOICE		BAD CHOICE	
Fruit Bowl	62	Chili Cheese Fries	681
Slow-Cooked Pot Roast	833	Artichoke & Pulled Crabmeat Casserole	1411
Strawberry Pie Slice	349	Key Lime Cheesecake	830
Total	**1244**	**Total**	**2922**

SILVER MINE SUBS. . . . . *SAVE 621 CALORIES !*

GOOD CHOICE		BAD CHOICE	
Fruit Cup, 113 g	80	Potato Salad, 156 g	270
Side Salad, 81g	11	Grilled Chicken Salad, 232 g	156
Broccoli and Cheese Soup, 250 g	160	Chili, 250 g	280
Pikes Peak Or Bust Sub, 8", 216 g	327	Silver Plume Sub, 8", 314 g	493
Total	**578**	**Total**	**1199**

SKYLINE CHILI . . . . *SAVE 1730 CALORIES !*

GOOD CHOICE		BAD CHOICE	
Plain Potato	310	5-Way Potato	950
Greek Salad	60	Southwest Chicken Salad	460
Chili Bean Bowl	270	Coney Bowl	870
Greek Chicken Wrap	510	Southwest Chicken Wrap	670
Total	**1150**	**Total**	**2880**

SONIC DRIVE-IN . . . . *SAVE 1450 CALORIES !*

GOOD CHOICE		BAD CHOICE	
Lo-Cal Diet Lime Limeade, 428 g	10	Iced Latté, Chocolate /Caramel, 351 g	260
Tots, 70 g	200	Onion Rings, 156 g	500
Corn Dog, 74 g	210	Ex-Long Chili Cheese Coney, 258 g	660
Diet Coke® Float/Blended Float, 348 g	220	Peanut Butter Malt, 434 g	670
Total	**640**	**Total**	**2090**

SOUPER SALAD . . . . *SAVE 730 CALORIES !*

GOOD CHOICE

Lemonade, Premium, 20 oz.	160
Roasted Vegetables Salad	20
French Onion Soup, 5 oz. bowl	40
Vegetable Lasagna	120
Jell-O, sugar free.	10
Total.	**350**

BAD CHOICE

Smoothie, Mango, 20 oz.	350
Ham & Macaroni Salad.	190
Chicken Enchilada Soup, 5 oz. bowl	180
Beef Taco, 2 oz.	200
Vanilla Pudding	160
Total	**1080**

SOUPLANTATION . . . . *SAVE 1120 CALORIES !*

GOOD CHOICE

Classic Greek Salad, 1 cup	120
Asian Ginger Broth, 1 cup	50
Oriental Noodles & Green Beans, 1 cup	240
Sugar Free Mousse, 1/2 cup	40
Total.	**.450**

BAD CHOICE

Cream Chipotle Salad, 1/2 cup	350
Cheese w/ Smoked Ham Soup, 1 cup	350
Chicken Tetrazzini, 1 cup	480
Caramel Apple Cobbler, 1/2 cup	390
Total	**1570**

STARBUCKS . . . . *SAVE 1240 CALORIES !*

GOOD CHOICE

Tazo® Awake™ Brewed Tea	0
Greek Yogurt Honey Parfait.	290
Starbucks® Perfect Oatmeal	140
Chocolate Mini Sparkle Doughnut	120
Total.	**550**

BAD CHOICE

Wht Choco Frappuccino® Crème	480
Dark Cherry Yogurt Parfait	310
Ssge, Egg & Chz on English Muffin	500
Raspberry Scone.	500
Total	**1790**

STEAK ESCAPE. . . . . *SAVE 454 CALORIES !*

GOOD CHOICE

Plain Potato, 392 g	246
Side Salad, 168 g	40
Vegetarian Sandwich, 252 g	311
Total.	**.597**

BAD CHOICE

Potatoes with Steak, 568 g	393
Side Salad with Steak, 316 g	187
Classic Italian Sub, 238 g	471
Total	**1051**

SUBWAY . . . . *SAVE 1365 CALORIES !*

GOOD CHOICE		BAD CHOICE	
Baked Lay's®, 32 g	130	Doritos Nacho Cheese, 50 g	250
Veggie Delite Salad, 300 g	50	Sweet Onion Chkn Teriyaki Salad, 413 g	200
Roasted Chicken Noodle Soup, 10 oz	80	Chili Con Carne, 10 oz	340
Veggie Delite Sandwich, 169 g	230	Double Meat Marinara w/cheese Sub	860
Apple Slices, 71 g	35	Apple Pie, 71 g	250
Total	**535**	**Total**	**1900**

SWISS CHALET . . . . *SAVE 1890 CALORIES !*

GOOD CHOICE		BAD CHOICE	
Side Garden Salad, 110 g	20	Grilled Chicken Caesar Salad, 407 g	680
Classic 1/4 Chicken Breast Skinless, 124 g	180	Classic Chkn Double Leg w/ Skin, 278 g	630
Chargrilled Veggie Burger, 113 g	110	Chargrilled Bacon Cheese Burger, 298 g	890
Total	**310**	**Total**	**2200**

TACO BELL . . . . *SAVE 770 CALORIES !*

GOOD CHOICE		BAD CHOICE	
Fiesta Taco Salad w/o Shell, 404 g	460	Chicken Ranch Taco Salad, 420 g	910
Burrito Supreme® - Steak, 248 g	380	Grilled Stuft Burrito - Beef, 325 g	700
Total	**840**	**Total**	**1610**

TACO CABANA . . . . *SAVE 1910 CALORIES !*

GOOD CHOICE		BAD CHOICE	
Shrimp Enchilada	190	Shrimp Tampico Quesadilla, regular	1450
Carne Guisada Dinner	840	Super Tex-Mex Dinner	1490
Total	**1030**	**Total**	**2940**

TACO DEL MAR . . . . *SAVE 1100 CALORIES !*

GOOD CHOICE	
Beans, whole pinto, 120 g	90
Soft Taco, chicken, 165 g	260
Cookie, Butter, 71 g	220
Total	**570**

BAD CHOICE	
Rice, 170 g	230
Fish Taco Salad, refried, 617 g	1040
Brownie, Oreo, 92 g	400
Total	**1670**

TACO JOHN'S . . . . *SAVE 1380 CALORIES !*

GOOD CHOICE	
Chili, 213 g	160
Crispy Taco, 92 g	180
Bean Burrito, 187 g	360
Giant Goldfish® Grahams, 14 g	70
Total	**770**

BAD CHOICE	
Potato Olés®, 201 g	600
Stuffed Grilled Taco, 211 g	560
Beef Grilled Burrito, 233 g	600
Choco Taco, 113 g	390
Total	**2150**

TACO MAYO . . . . *SAVE 1483 CALORIES !*

GOOD CHOICE	
Mexicali Rice	160
SalsaLITA Chicken Salad	278
SalsaLITA Chicken Burrito	325
Total	**763**

BAD CHOICE	
Potato Locos	586
Acapulco Salad - Steak	705
Double Smothered Chili Queso Burrito	955
Total	**2246**

TACO TIME . . . . *SAVE 1140 CALORIES !*

GOOD CHOICE	
Mexi-Rice, 4 oz.	80
Taco Salad, Chicken, 10 oz.	310
Enchilada, Chicken, 7 oz.	230
Churro, plain, 2 oz.	210
Total	**830**

BAD CHOICE	
Fries, Cheddar, 7 oz.	500
Tostada Delight Salad, Ground Beef, 9 oz.	490
Chicken B.L.T., 10 oz.	690
Crustos, 4 oz.	290
Total	**1970**

ORDER THE RIGHT MEAL

TACONE . . . . *SAVE 1600 CALORIES !*

GOOD CHOICE

Grilled Veggies + Feta, 113 g	170
Caesar Salad, 307 g	500
Tradewind Shrimp, 457 g	250
Orangabang, 539 g	360
Total.	**1280**

BAD CHOICE

Sweet Potato Fries, 109 g	190
Fiesta Salad, 310 g	340
Rotisserie Chicken, 595 g	830
Pink Flamingo, 658 g	520
Total	**2880**

TIM HORTON'S . . . . *SAVE 900 CALORIES !*

GOOD CHOICE

Tea w/ cream and sugar, 10 oz.	50
Hearty Vegetable Soup, 10 oz.	70
Egg, Cheese Sandwich 149 g	370
Oatmeal Raisin Spice Cookie, 52 g	220
Total.	**710**

BAD CHOICE

Iced Cappuccino, 12 oz.	300
Chili, 10 oz.	300
Sausage, Egg, Cheese Sandwich 191 g.	540
Cinnamon Roll- Frosted, 119 g	470
Total	**1610**

TOPZ . . . . *SAVE 869 CALORIES !*

GOOD CHOICE

Aero Onion Rings, 166 g	298
Small Dijon Deli Salad, 21 g	101
Garden Burger, 228 g	355
Low Fat Ice Cream w/ Choco Syrup, 162 g	255
Total.	**1009**

BAD CHOICE

Chocolate Banana Shake, 472 g	460
Chili Cheese Fries, 301 g	589
Chinese Chicken Salad, 392 g	322
1/4 lb. Black Angus Burger, 301 g	507
Total	**1878**

TROPICAL SMOOTHIE . . . . *SAVE 1121 CALORIES !*

GOOD CHOICE

Blue Lagoon™ Smoothie.	130
TSC Signature™ salad	349
Wasabi Roast Beef™ Wrap	374
Total.	**853**

BAD CHOICE

Caramel Cream™ Smoothie	591
Sesame Chicken™ Salad.	580
Sesame Chicken™ Wrap	803
Total	**1974**

UNA MAS . . . . *SAVE 1121 CALORIES !*

GOOD CHOICE		BAD CHOICE	
Strawberry Lemonade	.70	Horchata	480
Mexican Fried Rice	90	Rice and Beans	.240
Niño Burrito	403	Carnitas Burrito, The Works	.1560
Total	**563**	**Total**	**2280**

WAHOO'S FISH TACO . . . . *SAVE 936 CALORIES !*

GOOD CHOICE		BAD CHOICE	
Maui Onion Rings, 4	128	Baja Rolls, 3	168
Shrimp Salad	210	Carnitas Salad	580
Shrimp, Brown Rice, White Beans, Burrito	476	Carnitas, Wet Burrito	1002
Total	**.814**	**Total**	**1750**

WENDY'S . . . . *SAVE 1780 CALORIES !*

GOOD CHOICE		BAD CHOICE	
5 Piece Chicken Nugget	230	Sweet & Spicy Asian Boneless Wings	540
Side Salad	35	Chicken BLT Salad	.470
Grilled Chicken Go Wrap	250	Triple w/Everything and Cheese	.1030
Chocolate Frosty Small	.310	M&M's Twisted Frosty, Vanilla	560
Total	**820**	**Total**	**2600**

WHATABURGER . . . . *SAVE 2779 CALORIES !*

GOOD CHOICE		BAD CHOICE	
Coffee Decaf, Colombian, 473 g	.10	Malt, chocolate, 716 g	.1050
Fruit Chew, 26 g	80	French Fries, 128 g	480
Side Salad, 120 g	25	Chicken Strips Salad, 352 g	350
Justaburger®, 124 g	290	Whataburger®, Triple Meat, 492 g	.1120
Cookie, Sugar, 51 g	.210	Cinnamon Roll, 128 g	390
Total	**615**	**Total**	**3390**

WHITE CASTLE . . . . *SAVE 1712 CALORIES !*

GOOD CHOICE	
Iced Tea, Black Unsweetened, 30 g	0
Clam Strips, 128 g	128
Double White Castle, 98 g	240
Oatmeal Raisin Cookie, 38 g	160
Total.	**.528**

BAD CHOICE	
Chocolate Shake, 30 g	780
Onion Chips, 173 g	.670
Double Fish with Cheese, 164 g	.610
White Choco Macadamia Cookie, 38 g	.180
Total	**.2240**

WIENERSCHNITZEL . . . . *SAVE 1510 CALORIES !*

GOOD CHOICE	
Side Salad, 91 g	70
Corn Dog, 82 g	250
Kids Cone, 94 g	210
Total.	**.530**

BAD CHOICE	
Chili Cheese Fries, 231 g	540
Angus All Beef Pastrami Dog, 260 g	680
Banana Split, 450 g	820
Total	**.2040**

WINCHELL'S . . . . *SAVE 1280 CALORIES !*

GOOD CHOICE	
Hot Cocoa, 20 oz	440
Jalapeño Bagel, 113 g	250
Puffies w/ Vanilla Cream Filling, 50 g	150
Total.	**840**

BAD CHOICE	
Vanilla Caramel Cappuccino Chilla, 20 oz	980
Bacon & Cheddar on Plain Bagel, 151 g	440
Bear Claw, 184 g	700
Total	**.2120**

WING STREET . . . . *SAVE 490 CALORIES !*

GOOD CHOICE	
Baked Hot Wings, 2 pieces	.100
Tomato, Mushroom & Jalapeño Pizza, 87 g	150
Cinnamon Sticks, 2 pieces, 55 g	170
Total.	**420**

BAD CHOICE	
Fried Cheese Sticks (4 pcs), 119 g	380
Meat Lover's®, 113 g	330
Hershey's® Choco Dunkers®, 60 g	200
Total	**910**

YARD HOUSE . . . . *SAVE 4170 CALORIES !*

GOOD CHOICE		BAD CHOICE	
Caesar Salad	435	BBQ Chicken Salad	1665
Hawaiian Fresh Fish Healthy Dining	645	New York Steak	2425
Mango Sorbet	195	Macadamia Nut Cheesecake	1355
Total	**1275**	**Total**	**5445**

YOSHINOYAS . . . . *SAVE 1525 CALORIES !*

GOOD CHOICE		BAD CHOICE	
Vegetables	60	Rice	460
Chicken Only Bowl	255	Shrimp & Beef Bowl	1280
Flan	230	Chocolate Cake	330
Total	**545**	**Total**	**2070**

FAVORITE SODAS AND JUICE

SODA	CAL
7Up 100% Natural Flavors, 8 fl.oz.	100
Barq's Root Beer, 8 fl.oz.	111
Coca-Cola classic, 8 fl.oz.	97
Dr. Pepper, 8 fl.oz.	100
Mountain Dew, 8 fl.oz.	110
Pepsi, 8 fl.oz.	100
Pibb Xtra, 8 fl.oz.	97
Sprite, 8 fl.oz.	96
Sunkist Orange, 8 fl.oz	130

Diet

Diet Soda, 8 fl.oz.	0
Fresca, 8 fl.oz.	2

JUICE	CAL
Apple Juice, 8 fl.oz.	120
Fruit Punch, 8 fl.oz.	110
Orange Juice, 8 fl.oz.	110
Lemonade, 8 fl.oz.	110
Pink Lemonade, 8 fl.oz.	100

FAVORITE ALCOHOLIC DRINKS

BEERS	CAL
Light	
Amstel Light, 1 bottle	100
Bud Light, 12 fl oz	110
Coors Light, 12 fl oz	102
Corona Light, 1 bottle	105

Kirin Light, 12.2 fl oz	100
Michelob Ultra, 1 bottle	73
Miller Lite, 12 fl oz	96
Milwaukee's Best Light, 12.2 fl oz	98
Natural Light, 12 fl oz	95
Samuel Adams Light, 12 fl oz	119

FAVORITE ALCOHOLIC DRINKS

BEERS (CONT'D) . . . . CAL

Regular

Blue Moon, 12 fl oz	171
Budweiser , 12 fl oz	145
Corona Extra, 1 bottle	148
Guinness, Stout, 1 pint	170
Heineken, 1 bottle	140
Kirin, 12.2 fl oz	145
Miller Genuine Draft, 12 fl oz	143
Newcastle, 12 fl oz	140
Samuel Adams, 12 fl oz	180
Stella Artois, 11.2 fl oz	154

Non-Alcoholic

Beck's Non-Alcoholic, 12 fl oz	90
O'Douls, 12 fl oz	70

COCKTAILS . . . . CAL

Alexander, 1 cocktail	170
Black Russian, 1 cocktail	240
Bloody Mary, 1 cocktail	115
Bourbon & Soda, 1 cocktail	105
Daiquiri, 1 cocktail	113
Gin & Tonic, 1 cocktail	197
Grasshopper, 1 cocktail	222
High Ball, 1 cocktail	107
Lemon Drop Martini, 1 cocktail	150
Long Island Ice Tea, 1 cocktail	140
Mai Tai, 1 cocktail	264
Manhattan, 1 cocktail	136
Margarita, 1 cocktail	159
Martini, Vodka, 1 cocktail	210
Mint Julep, 1 cocktail	188
Mojito, 1 cocktail	100
Piña Colada, 1 cocktail	440
Rum and Coke, 1 cocktail	150
Sangria, 1 cocktail	165
Screwdriver, 1 cocktail	171
Seven and Seven, 1 cocktail	180
Singapore Sling, 1 cocktail	230
Tequila Sunrise, 1 cocktail	175
Tom Collins, 1 cocktail	156
Whiskey Sour, 1 cocktail	139
White Russian, 1 cocktail	253

LIQUEURS. . . . . CAL

99 Apples - 49.5% (99 prf), 1 oz.	72
Alize - 16.0% (32 prf), 1 oz.	103
Amaretto - 28.0% (56 prf), 1 oz.	110
Barenfang - 40.0% (80 prf), 1 oz.	103
Continental - 17.5% (35 proof), 1 oz.	85
Crème de Cassis - 20.0% (40 proof), 1 oz.	80
Crème de Coconut - 17.0% (34 proof), 1 oz.	103
Forbidden Fruit - 50.0% (100 proof),1 oz.	103
Godiva - 17.0% (34 proof),1 oz.	103
Jagermeister - 35.0% (70 proof), 1 oz.	103
Jubilee - 24.0% (48 proof), 1 oz.	72
Kahlua- 26.5% (53 proof), 1 oz.	90
Maui Blue Hawaiian - 15.0% (30 proof), 1 oz.	72
Midori - 23.0% (46 proof), 1 oz.	79
Sour Puss - 15.5% (31 proof), 1 oz.	103
Tequila Rose - 17.0% (34 proof), 1 oz.	69
Zwack - 43.0% (86 proof),1 oz.	87

LIQUORS. . . . . CAL

Brandy - 40.0% (80 proof), 1 oz.	69
Gin - 40.0% (80 proof), 1 oz.	69
Rum - 40.0% (80 proof), 1 oz.	69
Tequila - 40.0% (80 proof), 1 oz.	69
Vodka - 40.0% (80 proof), 1 oz.	69
Whiskey - 40.0% (80 proof), 1 oz.	69

SHOOTERS. . . . . CAL

Buttery Nipple, 1.5 fl oz	130
Chocolate Cake Shot, 1 shot	85
Fuzzy Navel, 1.5 fl oz	120
Kamikazi, 1.5 fl oz	150
Purple Hooter, 1.5 fl oz	90
Red-Headed Slut, 2 oz	164
Soco Lime, 2 oz	167
Vodka Lemon Drop, 1 oz	38
Washington Apple, 3 oz	140

WINE . . . . CAL

Dry Dessert Wine, 1 fl. oz.	45
Red Table Wine, 1 fl. oz.	25
Sweet Dessert Wine, 1 fl. oz.	47
White Table Wine, 1 fl. oz.	25

"The secret of health for both mind and body is not to mourn for the past, nor to worry about the future, but to live the present moment wisely and earnestly.**"**

~ Buddha

Chapter 20

How to Use the Journal Pages

These journal pages are an instrumental part of losing 10 pounds in 2 weeks because they help you monitor your weight, calorie intake, and calories burned through exercise. The best way to create a significant calorie deficit per day is to plan ahead and create a calorie "budget" for each meal and snack and determine how much exercise you need to burn additional calories. Anticipating how many calories you can "spend" at each meal takes the guesswork out of cooking and ordering off restaurant menus. For instance, if you have 400 calories to budget for lunch, you may decide to order a turkey sub with cheese and spend the whole amount, or you may opt for the veggie sub with no cheese and save 150 calories.

The journal pages also give you clues into how food, exercise and hydration factor into your mood and energy levels. You may find fascinating correlations between what and when you're eating and how great or lousy you're feeling. Plus, nothing is a better motivator for exercise than realizing how much more energy and stamina you have throughout the day when you've hit the gym or gone for a bike ride.

Another great benefit of a diet and fitness journal is it keeps you accountable. It's easy to let a 150-calorie cookie slip your mind, or to tell yourself you worked out for 30 minutes when it was really only 20, but those little white lies are much more difficult when you're recording everything in a journal throughout the day. You've likely put on extra weight by not holding yourself accountable in the past; this journal will help you break that bad habit and start keeping track of everything you eat, drink and do by way of exercise. It's the proven way to slim down faster!

Here is an explanation of the different components of the journal pages:

❶ DAILY NUTRITIONAL INTAKE: Record your daily intake of calories, fats and carbs for each meal and snack. Write down your totals for breakfast, lunch, dinner, and two snacks. Compare these totals to your nutritional intake goal from earlier in this book and see if you are meeting or going over your target amounts. There is also a column called "Other" that can be used to track intake of protein, fiber, sugar, sodium or another nutrient if you have special dietary concerns, such as high blood pressure or diabetes.

❷ WATER INTAKE: Strive for at least eight 8-ounce glasses of water per day. Check off a box for each glass you drink. If you drink water on a regular basis throughout the day, your metabolism works faster and better and you'll have more energy for exercise.

❸ DAILY NUMBER OF SERVINGS: At the end of each day, write down the number of servings you ate from each of the six major food groups. Eating a balanced diet is a big part of losing weight and keeping it off.

❹ VITAMINS & SUPPLEMENTS: Make note of the vitamins or supplements you are including in your program. When in doubt about specific vitamin recommendations, consult with a health care professional.

❺ DAILY GOAL: Write down a goal each day and try your best to stick to it. When you do meet your daily goal, check off the box and you can feel proud of your success!

❻ PHYSICAL ACTIVITY: Record all physical activity you do, including cardio, strength training, flexibility training, or a combination of all three. Record the duration, distance, pace, weight, sets, number of repetitions, and total calories burned.

❼ CALORIE CALCULATOR: This formula helps you find your Daily Net Calorie Gain or Loss for each day. Start with your Total Calorie Intake for that day, subtract the Total Calories Burned from physical activity to get Net Calories. Then, subtract your BMR (the number of calories your body burns at rest, calculated earlier in this book) to get your Daily Net Calorie Gain or Loss. Your goal is for this to be a negative number, meaning you created a calorie deficit, which is necessary to lose weight.

❽ ENERGY LEVEL: Document your daily overall energy by rating your energy levels from 1 to 6. Take note of how your energy correlates to the types of foods you have eaten that day. For example, if you notice that a little extra protein helps you get through your workout with more energy, incorporate lean meats in your diet. As you discover these relationships, make adjustments as needed to help you feel your best.

❾ MUSCLE GROUP WORKED: Document which of the 6 major muscle groups you work each day during exercise. Strive to include workouts that work your entire body, but also pay attention to how your body feels and give certain muscle groups sufficient rest to prevent injury.

Sample Journal Page

DIET JOURNAL

Day 1

DATE: Feb. 2   WEIGHT: 197

❶ BREAKFAST

BREAKFAST	Qty.	Calories	Fat	Carbs	Protein Other
Blueberry scone	1	400	17	55	5
Orange juice	12 oz.	110	0	26	2

SNACK

SNACK	Qty.	Calories	Fat	Carbs	Other

LUNCH

LUNCH	Qty.	Calories	Fat	Carbs	Other
Bagel w/turkey		490	4	70	30
American cheese	2	64	2	2	8
Baby carrots		100	0	24	3
Pepsi	12 oz.	180	0	45	0

SNACK

SNACK	Qty.	Calories	Fat	Carbs	Other
Apple slices and peanut butter		245	17	21	10

DINNER

DINNER	Qty.	Calories	Fat	Carbs	Other
Salmon	8 oz.	416	22	0	45
Wild rice		166	2	34	7
Broccoli		54	1	12	2
Crystal Light tea		5	0	0	0

DAILY INTAKE TOTALS:	2,230	65	289	112

❷ **☑ Water Intake**
# of 8 oz. glasses

☑ ☑ ☑
☑ ☑ ☑
☑ ☑ ☐

❸ **Daily # of Servings**

3	fruits	2	meats & beans
2	veggies	1	milk & dairy
3	grains	3	oils & sweets

❹ **Vitamins & Supplements:**

Calcium
Vitamin C

FITNESS JOURNAL

❺

DAILY GOAL: *Eat a high-protein dinner + work out for 90⁺ mins.*   **GOAL MET:** ☑

❻

CARDIOVASCULAR EXERCISE	Duration	Distance	Pace	Cal. Burned
Shooting the basketball	60 mins		medium	300
Jogging around my neighborhood	20 mins	1.5 mi	4.5 mph	205

STRENGTH TRAINING	Weight	Reps.	Sets	Cal. Burned
Bicep curls	25	3	36	20
Pull-ups		2	8	25
Push-ups		2	60	35

FLEXIBILITY, RELAXATION, MEDITATION	Duration	Cal. Burned
Stretching	10 mins	5

DAILY CALORIES BURNED: 590

❼

CALORIE CALCULATOR

2,230	−	590	=	1,640	−	1,979	=	−339
TOTAL CALORIE INTAKE		TOTAL CALORIES BURNED		NET CALORIES		BMR (Basal Metabolic Rate)		DAILY NET CALORIE GAIN OR LOSS

❽ Energy Level: 1 2 3 4 ⑤ 6

❾ Muscle Group Worked: ☑ arms ☑ chest ☐ back ☐ core ☑ thighs ☑ calves

Diet & Workout Notes:

Need more fiber during breakfast! Buy oatmeal. Do 45 minutes of cardio tomorrow.

Day 1

DATE: _____   WEIGHT: _____

BREAKFAST	Qty.	Calories	Fat	Carbs	Other
_____	____				
_____	____				
_____	____				
_____	____				
_____	____				

SNACK	Qty.	Calories	Fat	Carbs	Other
_____	____				
_____	____				

LUNCH	Qty.	Calories	Fat	Carbs	Other
_____	____				
_____	____				
_____	____				
_____	____				
_____	____				

SNACK	Qty.	Calories	Fat	Carbs	Other
_____	____				
_____	____				

DINNER	Qty.	Calories	Fat	Carbs	Other
_____	____				
_____	____				
_____	____				
_____	____				
_____	____				

DAILY INTAKE TOTALS:

☑ **Water Intake**
# of 8 oz. glasses
☐ ☐ ☐
☐ ☐ ☐
☐ ☐ ☐

Daily # of Servings

☐ fruits   ☐ meats & beans
☐ veggies   ☐ milk & dairy
☐ grains   ☐ oils & sweets

Vitamins & Supplements:
_____
_____
_____

FITNESS JOURNAL

DAILY GOAL: _____ GOAL MET: ☐

CARDIOVASCULAR EXERCISE

	Duration	Distance	Pace	Cal. Burned

STRENGTH TRAINING

	Weight	Reps.	Sets	Cal. Burned

FLEXIBILITY, RELAXATION, MEDITATION

	Duration	Cal. Burned

DAILY CALORIES BURNED: ☐

CALORIE CALCULATOR

	−		=		−		=	
TOTAL CALORIE INTAKE		TOTAL CALORIES BURNED		NET CALORIES		BMR (Basal Metabolic Rate)		DAILY NET CALORIE GAIN OR LOSS

Energy Level: 👎 1 2 3 4 5 6 👍

Muscle Group Worked: ☐ arms ☐ chest ☐ back ☐ core ☐ thighs ☐ calves

Diet & Workout Notes:

_____

_____

_____

_____

Day 2

DATE: _____   WEIGHT: _____

BREAKFAST	Qty.	Calories	Fat	Carbs	Other
_____	_____				
_____	_____				
_____	_____				
_____	_____				
_____	_____				

SNACK	Qty.	Calories	Fat	Carbs	Other
_____	_____				
_____	_____				

LUNCH	Qty.	Calories	Fat	Carbs	Other
_____	_____				
_____	_____				
_____	_____				
_____	_____				
_____	_____				

SNACK	Qty.	Calories	Fat	Carbs	Other
_____	_____				
_____	_____				

DINNER	Qty.	Calories	Fat	Carbs	Other
_____	_____				
_____	_____				
_____	_____				
_____	_____				
_____	_____				

DAILY INTAKE TOTALS:

☑ **Water Intake**
# of 8 oz. glasses

Daily # of Servings

fruits   meats & beans

veggies   milk & dairy

grains   oils & sweets

Vitamins & Supplements:
_____
_____
_____
_____

FITNESS JOURNAL

DAILY GOAL: _____ GOAL MET: ☐

CARDIOVASCULAR EXERCISE

	Duration	Distance	Pace	Cal. Burned
_____				
_____				
_____				
_____				

STRENGTH TRAINING

	Weight	Reps.	Sets	Cal. Burned
_____				
_____				
_____				
_____				
_____				
_____				
_____				
_____				

FLEXIBILITY, RELAXATION, MEDITATION

	Duration	Cal. Burned
_____		
_____		
_____		

DAILY CALORIES BURNED: _____

CALORIE CALCULATOR

_____ −	_____ =	_____ −	_____ =	_____
TOTAL CALORIE INTAKE	TOTAL CALORIES BURNED	NET CALORIES	BMR (Basal Metabolic Rate)	DAILY NET CALORIE GAIN OR LOSS

Energy Level: 1 2 3 4 5 6

Muscle Group Worked: ☐ arms ☐ chest ☐ back ☐ core ☐ thighs ☐ calves

Diet & Workout Notes:

_____
_____
_____
_____

Day 3

DATE: _____   WEIGHT: _____

BREAKFAST	Qty.	Calories	Fat	Carbs	Other
_____	_____				
_____	_____				
_____	_____				
_____	_____				
_____	_____				

SNACK	Qty.	Calories	Fat	Carbs	Other
_____	_____				
_____	_____				

LUNCH	Qty.	Calories	Fat	Carbs	Other
_____	_____				
_____	_____				
_____	_____				
_____	_____				
_____	_____				

SNACK	Qty.	Calories	Fat	Carbs	Other
_____	_____				
_____	_____				

DINNER	Qty.	Calories	Fat	Carbs	Other
_____	_____				
_____	_____				
_____	_____				
_____	_____				
_____	_____				

DAILY INTAKE TOTALS:

☑ **Water Intake**
# of 8 oz. glasses

Daily # of Servings

- fruits
- veggies
- grains
- meats & beans
- milk & dairy
- oils & sweets

Vitamins & Supplements:

_____

_____

_____

FITNESS JOURNAL

DAILY GOAL: _____ GOAL MET: ☐

🏃 CARDIOVASCULAR EXERCISE

	Duration	Distance	Pace	Cal. Burned
_____				
_____				
_____				
_____				

🧍 STRENGTH TRAINING

	Weight	Reps.	Sets	Cal. Burned
_____				
_____				
_____				
_____				
_____				
_____				
_____				
_____				

太 FLEXIBILITY, RELAXATION, MEDITATION

	Duration	Cal. Burned
_____		
_____		
_____		

DAILY CALORIES BURNED: _____

CALORIE CALCULATOR

_____	−	_____	=	_____	−	_____	=	_____
TOTAL CALORIE INTAKE		TOTAL CALORIES BURNED		NET CALORIES		BMR (Basal Metabolic Rate)		DAILY NET CALORIE GAIN OR LOSS

Energy Level:
👎 1   2   3   4   5   6 👍

Muscle Group Worked:
☐ arms ☐ chest ☐ back ☐ core ☐ thighs ☐ calves

Diet & Workout Notes:

_____

_____

_____

_____

Day 4

DATE: _____   WEIGHT: _____

BREAKFAST	Qty.	Calories	Fat	Carbs	Other
_____	___				
_____	___				
_____	___				
_____	___				
_____	___				

SNACK	Qty.	Calories	Fat	Carbs	Other
_____	___				
_____	___				

LUNCH	Qty.	Calories	Fat	Carbs	Other
_____	___				
_____	___				
_____	___				
_____	___				
_____	___				

SNACK	Qty.	Calories	Fat	Carbs	Other
_____	___				
_____	___				

DINNER	Qty.	Calories	Fat	Carbs	Other
_____	___				
_____	___				
_____	___				
_____	___				
_____	___				

DAILY INTAKE TOTALS:

☑ **Water Intake**
# of 8 oz. glasses

Daily # of Servings

- fruits
- veggies
- grains
- meats & beans
- milk & dairy
- oils & sweets

Vitamins & Supplements:

_____
_____
_____
_____

FITNESS JOURNAL

DAILY GOAL: _____ GOAL MET: ☐

🏃 CARDIOVASCULAR EXERCISE

	Duration	Distance	Pace	Cal. Burned
_____				
_____				
_____				
_____				

🏋 STRENGTH TRAINING

	Weight	Reps.	Sets	Cal. Burned
_____				
_____				
_____				
_____				
_____				
_____				
_____				
_____				

🧘 FLEXIBILITY, RELAXATION, MEDITATION

	Duration	Cal. Burned
_____		
_____		
_____		

DAILY CALORIES BURNED: ☐

CALORIE CALCULATOR

☐	–	☐	=	☐	–	☐	=	☐
TOTAL CALORIE INTAKE		TOTAL CALORIES BURNED		NET CALORIES		BMR (Basal Metabolic Rate)		DAILY NET CALORIE GAIN OR LOSS

Energy Level:
👎 1 2 3 4 5 6 👍

Muscle Group Worked:
☐ arms ☐ chest ☐ back ☐ core ☐ thighs ☐ calves

Diet & Workout Notes:

_____

_____

_____

_____

Day 5

DATE: _____   WEIGHT: _____

BREAKFAST	Qty.	Calories	Fat	Carbs	Other
_____	____				
_____	____				
_____	____				
_____	____				
_____	____				

SNACK	Qty.	Calories	Fat	Carbs	Other
_____	____				
_____	____				

LUNCH	Qty.	Calories	Fat	Carbs	Other
_____	____				
_____	____				
_____	____				
_____	____				
_____	____				

SNACK	Qty.	Calories	Fat	Carbs	Other
_____	____				
_____	____				

DINNER	Qty.	Calories	Fat	Carbs	Other
_____	____				
_____	____				
_____	____				
_____	____				
_____	____				
_____	____				

DAILY INTAKE TOTALS:

☑ **Water Intake**
# of 8 oz. glasses

Daily # of Servings

- fruits
- veggies
- grains
- meats & beans
- milk & dairy
- oils & sweets

Vitamins & Supplements:

_____
_____
_____
_____

FITNESS JOURNAL

DAILY GOAL: _____ GOAL MET: ☐

CARDIOVASCULAR EXERCISE

	Duration	Distance	Pace	Cal. Burned

STRENGTH TRAINING

	Weight	Reps.	Sets	Cal. Burned

FLEXIBILITY, RELAXATION, MEDITATION

	Duration	Cal. Burned

DAILY CALORIES BURNED: ☐

CALORIE CALCULATOR

TOTAL CALORIE INTAKE	−	TOTAL CALORIES BURNED	=	NET CALORIES	−	BMR (Basal Metabolic Rate)	=	DAILY NET CALORIE GAIN OR LOSS

Energy Level: 1 2 3 4 5 6

Muscle Group Worked: ☐ arms ☐ chest ☐ back ☐ core ☐ thighs ☐ calves

Diet & Workout Notes:

_____
_____
_____
_____

Day 6

DATE: _____   WEIGHT: _____

BREAKFAST	Qty.	Calories	Fat	Carbs	Other
_____	_____				
_____	_____				
_____	_____				
_____	_____				
_____	_____				

SNACK	Qty.	Calories	Fat	Carbs	Other
_____	_____				
_____	_____				

LUNCH	Qty.	Calories	Fat	Carbs	Other
_____	_____				
_____	_____				
_____	_____				
_____	_____				
_____	_____				

SNACK	Qty.	Calories	Fat	Carbs	Other
_____	_____				
_____	_____				

DINNER	Qty.	Calories	Fat	Carbs	Other
_____	_____				
_____	_____				
_____	_____				
_____	_____				
_____	_____				

DAILY INTAKE TOTALS:

☑ **Water Intake**
# of 8 oz. glasses

☐ ☐ ☐
☐ ☐ ☐
☐ ☐ ☐

Daily # of Servings

fruits
veggies
grains
meats & beans
milk & dairy
oils & sweets

Vitamins & Supplements:

_____
_____
_____

FITNESS JOURNAL

DAILY GOAL: _____ GOAL MET: ☐

CARDIOVASCULAR EXERCISE

	Duration	Distance	Pace	Cal. Burned

STRENGTH TRAINING

	Weight	Reps.	Sets	Cal. Burned

FLEXIBILITY, RELAXATION, MEDITATION

	Duration	Cal. Burned

DAILY CALORIES BURNED:

CALORIE CALCULATOR

TOTAL CALORIE INTAKE	−	TOTAL CALORIES BURNED	=	NET CALORIES	−	BMR (Basal Metabolic Rate)	=	DAILY NET CALORIE GAIN OR LOSS

Energy Level: 1 2 3 4 5 6

Muscle Group Worked: ☐ arms ☐ chest ☐ back ☐ core ☐ thighs ☐ calves

Diet & Workout Notes:

_____

_____

_____

_____

Day 7

DATE: _____   WEIGHT: _____

BREAKFAST	Qty.	Calories	Fat	Carbs	Other
_____	___				
_____	___				
_____	___				
_____	___				
_____	___				

SNACK	Qty.	Calories	Fat	Carbs	Other
_____	___				
_____	___				

LUNCH	Qty.	Calories	Fat	Carbs	Other
_____	___				
_____	___				
_____	___				
_____	___				
_____	___				

SNACK	Qty.	Calories	Fat	Carbs	Other
_____	___				
_____	___				

DINNER	Qty.	Calories	Fat	Carbs	Other
_____	___				
_____	___				
_____	___				
_____	___				
_____	___				

DAILY INTAKE TOTALS:

☑ **Water Intake**
# of 8 oz. glasses

Daily # of Servings

☐ fruits   ☐ meats & beans
☐ veggies   ☐ milk & dairy
☐ grains   ☐ oils & sweets

Vitamins & Supplements:
_____
_____
_____
_____

FITNESS JOURNAL

DAILY GOAL: _____ GOAL MET: ☐

🏃 CARDIOVASCULAR EXERCISE

	Duration	Distance	Pace	Cal. Burned
_____				
_____				
_____				
_____				

🏋 STRENGTH TRAINING

	Weight	Reps.	Sets	Cal. Burned
_____				
_____				
_____				
_____				
_____				
_____				
_____				
_____				

🧘 FLEXIBILITY, RELAXATION, MEDITATION

	Duration	Cal. Burned
_____		
_____		
_____		

DAILY CALORIES BURNED: _____

CALORIE CALCULATOR

_____	−	_____	=	_____	−	_____	=	_____
TOTAL CALORIE INTAKE		TOTAL CALORIES BURNED		NET CALORIES		BMR (Basal Metabolic Rate)		DAILY NET CALORIE GAIN OR LOSS

Energy Level: 👎 1 2 3 4 5 6 👍

Muscle Group Worked: ☐ arms ☐ chest ☐ back ☐ core ☐ thighs ☐ calves

Diet & Workout Notes:

_____

_____

_____

_____

Day 8

DATE: _____   WEIGHT: _____

BREAKFAST	Qty.	Calories	Fat	Carbs	Other
_____	_____				
_____	_____				
_____	_____				
_____	_____				
_____	_____				

SNACK	Qty.	Calories	Fat	Carbs	Other
_____	_____				
_____	_____				

LUNCH	Qty.	Calories	Fat	Carbs	Other
_____	_____				
_____	_____				
_____	_____				
_____	_____				
_____	_____				

SNACK	Qty.	Calories	Fat	Carbs	Other
_____	_____				
_____	_____				

DINNER	Qty.	Calories	Fat	Carbs	Other
_____	_____				
_____	_____				
_____	_____				
_____	_____				
_____	_____				

DAILY INTAKE TOTALS:

☑ **Water Intake**
# of 8 oz. glasses

☐ ☐ ☐
☐ ☐ ☐
☐ ☐ ☐

Daily # of Servings

fruits   meats & beans
veggies   milk & dairy
grains   oils & sweets

Vitamins & Supplements:

_____
_____
_____

FITNESS JOURNAL

DAILY GOAL: _____ GOAL MET: ☐

CARDIOVASCULAR EXERCISE

	Duration	Distance	Pace	Cal. Burned
_____				
_____				
_____				
_____				

STRENGTH TRAINING

	Weight	Reps.	Sets	Cal. Burned
_____				
_____				
_____				
_____				
_____				
_____				
_____				
_____				

FLEXIBILITY, RELAXATION, MEDITATION

	Duration	Cal. Burned
_____		
_____		
_____		

DAILY CALORIES BURNED: _____

CALORIE CALCULATOR

_____	−	_____	=	_____	−	_____	=	_____
TOTAL CALORIE INTAKE		TOTAL CALORIES BURNED		NET CALORIES		BMR (Basal Metabolic Rate)		DAILY NET CALORIE GAIN OR LOSS

Energy Level: 👎 1 2 3 4 5 6 👍

Muscle Group Worked: ☐ arms ☐ chest ☐ back ☐ core ☐ thighs ☐ calves

Diet & Workout Notes:

_____

_____

_____

_____

Day 9

DATE: _____   WEIGHT: _____

🍎 BREAKFAST

	Qty.	Calories	Fat	Carbs	Other
_____	_____				
_____	_____				
_____	_____				
_____	_____				
_____	_____				

🥤 SNACK

	Qty.	Calories	Fat	Carbs	Other
_____	_____				
_____	_____				

🥪 LUNCH

	Qty.	Calories	Fat	Carbs	Other
_____	_____				
_____	_____				
_____	_____				
_____	_____				
_____	_____				

🍇 SNACK

	Qty.	Calories	Fat	Carbs	Other
_____	_____				
_____	_____				

🍽 DINNER

	Qty.	Calories	Fat	Carbs	Other
_____	_____				
_____	_____				
_____	_____				
_____	_____				
_____	_____				

DAILY INTAKE TOTALS:

☑ **Water Intake**
# of 8 oz. glasses

☐ ☐ ☐
☐ ☐ ☐
☐ ☐ ☐

Daily # of Servings

▢ fruits	▢ meats & beans	
▢ veggies	▢ milk & dairy	
▢ grains	▢ oils & sweets	

Vitamins & Supplements:

_____

_____

_____

FITNESS JOURNAL

DAILY GOAL: _____ GOAL MET: ☐

CARDIOVASCULAR EXERCISE

	Duration	Distance	Pace	Cal. Burned
_____				
_____				
_____				
_____				

STRENGTH TRAINING

	Weight	Reps.	Sets	Cal. Burned
_____				
_____				
_____				
_____				
_____				
_____				
_____				
_____				

FLEXIBILITY, RELAXATION, MEDITATION

	Duration	Cal. Burned
_____		
_____		
_____		

DAILY CALORIES BURNED: _____

CALORIE CALCULATOR

_____	−	_____	=	_____	−	_____	=	_____
TOTAL CALORIE INTAKE		TOTAL CALORIES BURNED		NET CALORIES		BMR (Basal Metabolic Rate)		DAILY NET CALORIE GAIN OR LOSS

Energy Level: 👎 1 2 3 4 5 6 👍

Muscle Group Worked:
☐ arms ☐ chest ☐ back ☐ core ☐ thighs ☐ calves

Diet & Workout Notes:

_____

_____

_____

_____

Day 10

DATE: _____   WEIGHT: _____

🍎 BREAKFAST	Qty.	Calories	Fat	Carbs	Other
_____	_____				
_____	_____				
_____	_____				
_____	_____				
_____	_____				

✚ SNACK	Qty.	Calories	Fat	Carbs	Other
_____	_____				
_____	_____				

🍔 LUNCH	Qty.	Calories	Fat	Carbs	Other
_____	_____				
_____	_____				
_____	_____				
_____	_____				
_____	_____				

🍇 SNACK	Qty.	Calories	Fat	Carbs	Other
_____	_____				
_____	_____				

🥄 DINNER	Qty.	Calories	Fat	Carbs	Other
_____	_____				
_____	_____				
_____	_____				
_____	_____				
_____	_____				

DAILY INTAKE TOTALS:

☑ **Water Intake**
# of 8 oz. glasses

▢ ▢ ▢
▢ ▢ ▢
▢ ▢ ▢

Daily # of Servings

☐ fruits   ☐ meats & beans
☐ veggies   ☐ milk & dairy
☐ grains   ☐ oils & sweets

Vitamins & Supplements:

_____
_____
_____
_____

FITNESS JOURNAL

DAILY GOAL: _____ GOAL MET: ☐

🏃 CARDIOVASCULAR EXERCISE

	Duration	Distance	Pace	Cal. Burned
_____				
_____				
_____				
_____				

🏋 STRENGTH TRAINING

	Weight	Reps.	Sets	Cal. Burned
_____				
_____				
_____				
_____				
_____				
_____				
_____				
_____				

方 FLEXIBILITY, RELAXATION, MEDITATION

	Duration	Cal. Burned
_____		
_____		
_____		

DAILY CALORIES BURNED: _____

CALORIE CALCULATOR

_____	−	_____	=	_____	−	_____	=	_____
TOTAL CALORIE INTAKE		TOTAL CALORIES BURNED		NET CALORIES		BMR (Basal Metabolic Rate)		DAILY NET CALORIE GAIN OR LOSS

Energy Level: 👎 1 2 3 4 5 6 👍

Muscle Group Worked: ☐ arms ☐ chest ☐ back ☐ core ☐ thighs ☐ calves

Diet & Workout Notes:

_____
_____
_____
_____

Day 11

DATE: _____   WEIGHT: _____

BREAKFAST	Qty.	Calories	Fat	Carbs	Other
_____	_____				
_____	_____				
_____	_____				
_____	_____				
_____	_____				

SNACK	Qty.	Calories	Fat	Carbs	Other
_____	_____				
_____	_____				

LUNCH	Qty.	Calories	Fat	Carbs	Other
_____	_____				
_____	_____				
_____	_____				
_____	_____				
_____	_____				

SNACK	Qty.	Calories	Fat	Carbs	Other
_____	_____				
_____	_____				

DINNER	Qty.	Calories	Fat	Carbs	Other
_____	_____				
_____	_____				
_____	_____				
_____	_____				
_____	_____				

DAILY INTAKE TOTALS:

☑ **Water Intake**
# of 8 oz. glasses

Daily # of Servings

fruits   meats & beans
veggies   milk & dairy
grains   oils & sweets

Vitamins & Supplements:

_____
_____
_____
_____

FITNESS JOURNAL

DAILY GOAL: _____   GOAL MET: ☐

🏃 CARDIOVASCULAR EXERCISE

	Duration	Distance	Pace	Cal. Burned

🏋 STRENGTH TRAINING

	Weight	Reps.	Sets	Cal. Burned

🧘 FLEXIBILITY, RELAXATION, MEDITATION

	Duration	Cal. Burned

DAILY CALORIES BURNED: _____

CALORIE CALCULATOR

TOTAL CALORIE INTAKE	−	TOTAL CALORIES BURNED	=	NET CALORIES	−	BMR (Basal Metabolic Rate)	=	DAILY NET CALORIE GAIN OR LOSS

Energy Level: 👎 1   2   3   4   5   6 👍

Muscle Group Worked: ☐ arms ☐ chest ☐ back ☐ core ☐ thighs ☐ calves

Diet & Workout Notes:

_____
_____
_____
_____

Day 12

DATE: _____   WEIGHT: _____

BREAKFAST	Qty.	Calories	Fat	Carbs	Other
_____	____				
_____	____				
_____	____				
_____	____				
_____	____				

SNACK	Qty.	Calories	Fat	Carbs	Other
_____	____				
_____	____				

LUNCH	Qty.	Calories	Fat	Carbs	Other
_____	____				
_____	____				
_____	____				
_____	____				
_____	____				

SNACK	Qty.	Calories	Fat	Carbs	Other
_____	____				
_____	____				

DINNER	Qty.	Calories	Fat	Carbs	Other
_____	____				
_____	____				
_____	____				
_____	____				
_____	____				

DAILY INTAKE TOTALS:

☑ **Water Intake**
# of 8 oz. glasses

Daily # of Servings

fruits		meats & beans	
veggies		milk & dairy	
grains		oils & sweets	

Vitamins & Supplements:
_____
_____
_____
_____

FITNESS JOURNAL

DAILY GOAL: _____ GOAL MET: ☐

🏃 CARDIOVASCULAR EXERCISE

	Duration	Distance	Pace	Cal. Burned
_____				
_____				
_____				
_____				

🏋 STRENGTH TRAINING

	Weight	Reps.	Sets	Cal. Burned
_____				
_____				
_____				
_____				
_____				
_____				
_____				
_____				

🤸 FLEXIBILITY, RELAXATION, MEDITATION

	Duration	Cal. Burned
_____		
_____		
_____		

DAILY CALORIES BURNED: ☐

CALORIE CALCULATOR

☐ − ☐ = ☐ − ☐ = ☐

| TOTAL CALORIE INTAKE | | TOTAL CALORIES BURNED | | NET CALORIES | | BMR (Basal Metabolic Rate) | | DAILY NET CALORIE GAIN OR LOSS |

Energy Level: 👎 1 2 3 4 5 6 👍

Muscle Group Worked: ☐ arms ☐ chest ☐ back ☐ core ☐ thighs ☐ calves

Diet & Workout Notes:

_____
_____
_____
_____

Day 13

DATE: _____   WEIGHT: _____

BREAKFAST	Qty.	Calories	Fat	Carbs	Other

SNACK	Qty.	Calories	Fat	Carbs	Other

LUNCH	Qty.	Calories	Fat	Carbs	Other

SNACK	Qty.	Calories	Fat	Carbs	Other

DINNER	Qty.	Calories	Fat	Carbs	Other

DAILY INTAKE TOTALS:

☑ **Water Intake**
# of 8 oz. glasses

Daily # of Servings

fruits   meats & beans
veggies   milk & dairy
grains   oils & sweets

Vitamins & Supplements:

_____

_____

_____

_____

FITNESS JOURNAL

DAILY GOAL: _____ **GOAL MET:** ☐

🏃 CARDIOVASCULAR EXERCISE

	Duration	Distance	Pace	Cal. Burned

🏋 STRENGTH TRAINING

	Weight	Reps.	Sets	Cal. Burned

🧘 FLEXIBILITY, RELAXATION, MEDITATION

	Duration	Cal. Burned

DAILY CALORIES BURNED: ☐

CALORIE CALCULATOR

☐ − ☐ = ☐ − ☐ = ☐

TOTAL CALORIE INTAKE	TOTAL CALORIES BURNED	NET CALORIES	BMR (Basal Metabolic Rate)	DAILY NET CALORIE GAIN OR LOSS

Energy Level: 👎 1 2 3 4 5 6 👍

Muscle Group Worked: ☐ arms ☐ chest ☐ back ☐ core ☐ thighs ☐ calves

Diet & Workout Notes:

_____
_____
_____
_____

Day 14

DATE: _____   WEIGHT: _____

🍎 BREAKFAST	Qty.	Calories	Fat	Carbs	Other
_____	___				
_____	___				
_____	___				
_____	___				
_____	___				

SNACK	Qty.	Calories	Fat	Carbs	Other
_____	___				
_____	___				

LUNCH	Qty.	Calories	Fat	Carbs	Other
_____	___				
_____	___				
_____	___				
_____	___				
_____	___				

SNACK	Qty.	Calories	Fat	Carbs	Other
_____	___				
_____	___				

DINNER	Qty.	Calories	Fat	Carbs	Other
_____	___				
_____	___				
_____	___				
_____	___				
_____	___				

DAILY INTAKE TOTALS:

☑ **Water Intake**
# of 8 oz. glasses

Daily # of Servings

	fruits		meats & beans
	veggies		milk & dairy
	grains		oils & sweets

Vitamins & Supplements:

_____

_____

_____

_____

FITNESS JOURNAL

DAILY GOAL: _____   **GOAL MET:** ☐

CARDIOVASCULAR EXERCISE

	Duration	Distance	Pace	Cal. Burned

STRENGTH TRAINING

	Weight	Reps.	Sets	Cal. Burned

FLEXIBILITY, RELAXATION, MEDITATION

	Duration	Cal. Burned

DAILY CALORIES BURNED: _____

CALORIE CALCULATOR

_____	−	_____	=	_____	−	_____	=	_____
TOTAL CALORIE INTAKE		TOTAL CALORIES BURNED		NET CALORIES		BMR (Basal Metabolic Rate)		DAILY NET CALORIE GAIN OR LOSS

Energy Level: 1   2   3   4   5   6

Muscle Group Worked: ☐ arms   ☐ chest   ☐ back   ☐ core   ☐ thighs   ☐ calves

Diet & Workout Notes:

_____

_____

_____

_____

“Every human being is the author of his own health or disease. **”**

~ Buddha

Chapter 21

After the 2 Weeks

Congratulations, you made it through the 2 weeks! But what happens now? This chapter is going to cover the ways to maintain your weight loss and continue to lose even more weight — but first, you should celebrate your weight-loss accomplishments! Remember, use what you've learned in this book and celebrate without bingeing or indulging in a high-calorie meal. Healthy celebrations include going to a concert or sporting event, seeing a movie with a loved one, shopping for a new item of clothing to fit your slimmed-down shape, or treating yourself to a kitchen appliance you've had your eye on. If the reward helps you continue to lose weight after the 2 weeks, even better!

After you've sufficiently rewarded yourself for a job well done, it's time to think longer-term. Do you want to continue losing weight with this diet and fitness program? Well, why not? If you followed the food and exercise tips, tricks and secrets here you lost up to 10 pounds in a short amount of time without feeling stressed, starved or deprived. And after 2 weeks, these behaviors have had enough time to become real habits and lifestyle changes. So why stop now?

There are a few things to be aware of beyond the 2 weeks, however. For one, you may hit a point where your weight loss slows down from 2 pounds a week to 1 pound to even less. This is perfectly normal. Your body is slimming down, you have less weight and body fat to lose, and you are growing accustomed to eating less and exercising more. Consider getting a trainer who can help you mix up your routine, use new machines, and try new techniques you may never have considered. When you do the same exercises or strength training workout, you're firing the same muscle fibers again and again — and they begin to adapt. You may also need to work out longer to keep losing weight. But don't worry — as you build muscle and lose fat, your body will automatically burn more calories when it's at rest.

But truly, the greatest thing you'll find about the *Lose Up To 10 Pounds in 2 Weeks* program is that exercising and eating right become a way of life! Plopping down on the couch with a bag of chips won't seem appealing to you anymore. And your body will have become used to eating smaller meals, so pigging out on half a pizza won't be on your mind.

Just don't lose your focus, stop watching your portion sizes, or get lazy with exercise. Read on for some great ways to enjoy your success but keep losing weight while sticking to your new, healthy, happy lifestyle.

Start thinking of yourself as thin

Sadly, many people who slim down still view themselves as their former, fatter selves. They wear the same clothes they wore when they were heavier or save a place in their closets for their "fat" clothes. Many overweight people shy away from wearing bright colors that draw attention to problem areas and still end up dressing in all black after they lose weight. But now is the time to embrace change and show off your hard work! Invest in a few new pieces and feel proud wearing them. Not only are you rewarding yourself, you'll look better, too. Wearing clothing that is too big for you isn't flattering and will only hide your flatter stomach and more defined arms and legs. And do some closet spring cleaning, too. Anything dowdy or oversized or out of shape can be donated to charity. Some people hold on to all their old clothes because they're afraid they'll gain the weight back, but getting rid of them means you're saying goodbye to the old you who sat on the couch with a bowl of ice cream every night. This new you exercises, eats right throughout the week, and celebrates a healthy, thinner figure. Just don't go on a shopping spree if you're planning to lose more weight (and you should be!). Wait until you're down 2 full sizes to splurge on a new wardrobe.

Revamp your daily routine to include fitness

So, how many days a week are you going to need to exercise to maintain or increase your weight loss after the 2 weeks of this program are up? Consider that the men and women of the National Weight Control Registry (a roster of more than 6,000 participants who, on average, have lost 66 pounds and kept them off for five and a half years), report exercising for an average of 60 to 75 minutes daily. If you are not the type of person who enjoys going to a gym you'll need to integrate other forms of calorie-burning activities into your life. For instance, vacuuming for one hour burns 220 calories, grocery shopping requires 180 calories, and an afternoon of gardening, sweeping and raking leaves expends 270 calories. If your home or office has stairs, walking up them in a moderate manner for 15 minutes burns 120 calories. Need a room in your house painted? Do it yourself and burn 340 calories an hour. Live in an area with snow? You've hit the jackpot — shoveling snow for an hour burns 600 calories. Combining a few of these forms of aerobic activity is the equivalent of spending a couple of hours at the gym.

Make new friends who also care about healthy living

If you've joined a gym or fitness class or group, you have ample opportunities to make new friends, and the best part is, these are people who care about being healthy and staying slim. Losing weight also opens doors to more confidence and many times, a new social life. Accept more invitations to parties and get-togethers; wear something that makes you feel amazing and that shows off your hard work. Being around people who share your interest in eating well and being healthy, as well as people who praise your weight loss, will keep you motivated to keep working hard.

Must have a treat? Keep it reasonable

If you really want to enjoy a treat in the form of food, keep it under 250 calories. A small sundae or amazing cupcake will do the trick. Just consciously remind yourself that this is a treat at the end of your hard work and not an invitation to go back to your old bad habits. This is a one-time celebration and not a weekly event.

Beat the weight-loss plateau

Naturally, the same diet and workout aren't going to produce the same results week after week. There are many ways to break through the plateaus you'll inevitably encounter. Let's say you have been doing cardio 5 days a week for 45 minutes; either add an extra 15 minutes to a few workouts, or else turn a normal session into an interval session just by interspersing 30- to 60-second bursts of speed and intensity every few minutes. Or, break through a plateau by changing up your meal routine. For instance, try eating a bigger lunch with more fiber and a smaller dinner. This can help take advantage of when your metabolism is faster during the day.

Document your progress with photos and measurements

The scale may not always accurately reflect your weight loss, considering that muscle greatly outweighs fat and water weight can be a factor, as well. The best way to document your progress is with photos (take them in a similar swimsuit each time) and by measuring yourself around the hips, thighs, stomach, chest, and arms. Losing inches (and pants and dress sizes) are the true test of your weight-loss success. And, seeing your new, slimmer self reflected in photos is one of the best testaments to how well this program has worked for you. When you feel like giving up or going back to your old ways, you can look at your Before and After photos and feel fantastic about how far you've come and how much weight you've lost all over. This confidence and pride are what keeps you going beyond the 2 weeks.

Stave off boredom

One common excuse for abandoning a workout or weight-loss program is boredom. Naturally, people get sick of the same gym grind or meal plan. When boredom starts to threaten your weight loss, it's time to introduce a new form of exercise or try one that never gets dull. Yoga, for instance, is a fantastic full-body workout and is a practice that is ever-evolving. Because there's always a new level of intensity or difficulty to reach, your body will never get complacent and you won't get bored. Or try taking up something that takes a long time to master, such as surfing, which is a great full-body workout — and fun, too!

The same concept goes for the foods you eat, too. Although a minority of people say they like the routine of eating the same thing at every meal, most people get bored and eventually succumb to cravings. Change up your go-to low-calorie meals in easy ways. Swap in grilled salmon for chicken in a salad; add shredded chicken and avocado to a bowl of soup; experiment with a new vegetable on the side of your dinner.

Update your music playlist every month

Music inspires you to get moving and keep moving. A great playlist keeps your energy up, but, just like anything, you will get bored if you're listening to the same songs day in and day out. It's a great idea to make separate playlists for different workouts of different intensities; for example, a super-fast set of songs for running, interval training and weight lifting, a slower set for jogging, and a relaxing, calming set for stretching and cooling down. Try varying the songs on each playlist every month. Check on your local radio stations' websites for what's new, or visit ShapeMagazine.com — they offer great monthly playlists for up-tempo workouts, and you can click right through to purchase the songs on iTunes.

Calculate your new daily calorie allowance

Now that you've lost up to 10 pounds, you may be ready to simply maintain your weight, or, you may be interested in losing even more. To do that, you need to calculate your new BMR (it changes as you lose weight) and new daily calorie allowance. That is the number of calories you'd need to eat each day to maintain your current weight. If you want to lose more weight, you should create another Calorie deficit, in the same way you did throughout this program.

The following equation uses your new BMR and factors in activity level:

To calculate your new BMR:

Women BMR = 655 + (4.3 x weight in pounds) + (4.7 x height in inches) - (4.7 x age in years)

Men BMR = 66 + (6.3 x weight in pounds) + (12.9 x height in inches) - (6.8 x age in years)

To find daily calorie allowance, choose the appropriate activity level and multiply your BMR accordingly.

Sedentary (little or no exercise):

Calorie-Calculation = BMR x 1.2

Lightly active (light exercise/activity 1-3 days/week):

Calorie-Calculation = BMR x 1.375

Moderately active (moderate exercise/activity 3-5 days/week):

Calorie-Calculation = BMR x 1.55

Very active (hard exercise/activity 6-7 days a week):

Calorie-Calculation = BMR x 1.725

Extra active (very hard exercise/activity, physical job or sports conditioning):

Calorie-Calculation = BMR x 1.9

The result of this calculation is the number of calories you can eat every day and maintain your current weight. If you want to lose more weight, reduce your calories to a number below your maintenance level. Just keep in mind that, according to the American College of Sports Medicine, calorie intake should never drop below 1,200 calories per day for women or 1,800 calories per day for men. Even those amounts are incredibly low. Keep your calories at a level that allows you to feel full and gives you enough energy for exercise.

Do what works for others

An important part of observing National Weight Control Registry members is determining how they manage to keep the weight off when such a huge majority of dieters fail to do so. In the end, there are 3 main factors that members continue to report again and again, which this book has already highlighted. Stick with these moving forward and you're sure to keep the weight off and lose even more. In order to maintain their weight loss, NWCR members:

- 78% eat breakfast every day
- 62% watch less than 10 hours of TV per week
- 90% exercise, on average, about 1 hour per day

Get your family and friends involved in your new lifestyle

The only way to maintain this new, healthier way of life is to get the people closest to you onboard, as well. That means being active with your family and friends. If you have kids, take up an activity that you can all do together, such as horseback riding, skiing, cycling, surfing or even yoga. If you have very young children, a game of tag is enough to get you all active and moving together.

Invite your friends to be active with you as well. Most people will be excited and willing to try a new activity with you, especially if they have witnessed your weight-loss success firsthand.

Your family and friends should also join you in your efforts to eat low-calorie, low-fat meals as often as possible. Try adding shredded vegetables, such as carrots, squash or zucchini, into pasta sauces or substituting meatless products into things like burritos and omelets — your fellow diners will never know the difference! Serve healthy desserts, such as fresh fruit with low-fat whipped topping, and your family will start to crave the same healthy foods that are helping you lose weight.

Don't stop using a diet and fitness journal!

Losing weight is one thing but keeping it off is another. Unfortunately, most people who successfully lose weight end up putting it, plus more, back on. A government review of numerous weight-loss studies found that two-thirds of dieters gain all the weight back within a year. But why does it happen and how can you avoid being part of that statistic?

For one, people get lazy once they've lost weight. They stop doing what worked for them. They stop monitoring their portion sizes and stop keeping a food and fitness journal. Don't forget how easy it is for the calories from a handful of M&M's at work or finishing your child's hotdog at a baseball game to creep in.

Don't stop keeping your diet and fitness journal just because this program is over. You can easily continue using the same secrets and methods for losing even more weight. Be sure to get a new journal before you've completely filled out the 2 weeks of journal pages in this book — that way you won't miss even a day! Try the *Ultimate Pocket Diet Journal*, one of the best-selling diet journals on the market. Also, you should keep a calorie-counting tool handy for when you dine out and items don't offer nutritional information. A great book is the portable, pocket-size *Complete Calorie, Fat & Carb Counter*, which provides calories, fat, carbs, fiber and protein for menu items from more than 500 fast-food chains, restaurants, and popular food brands.

Studies have shown again and again that keeping a diet and workout journal is one of the most effective tools for weight loss there is. Your success with this program should have confirmed that fact for you. So don't stop making great choices and writing them down!

> "Knowledge comes by eyes always open and working hands; and there is no knowledge that is not power."

~ Ralph Waldo Emerson

Chapter 22

Nutrition Facts

This section is a great resource for nutritional information on foods you may want to select for your fitness and weight-loss program. It provides calories per serving, as well as the content in grams for fat, protein, carbohydrates, and fiber.

To use this section, look up a food item and its corresponding information. Then, log this data in your journal so that you can track your daily totals.

NUTRITION FACTS

FOOD ITEM	Serving Size	Cal	Fat	Prtn	Cbs	Fbr
A						
Alcohol, 100 proof	1 fl.oz.	82	0	0	0	0
Alcohol, 86 proof	1 fl.oz.	70	0	0	0	0
Alcohol, 90 proof	1 fl.oz.	73	0	0	0	0
Alcohol, 94 proof	1 fl.oz.	76	0	0	0	0
Alcohol, dessert wine, dry	1 glass	157	0	0	12	0
Alcohol, dessert wine, sweet	1 glass	165	0	0	14	0
Alcohol, liquors	1 fl.oz.	107	0	0	11	0
Alcohol, piña colada	8 fl.oz.	440	5	1	57	0
Alfalfa seeds	1 tbsp	1	0	0	0	0
Allspice, ground	1 tsp	5	0	0	1	0
Almond butter, w/ salt	1 tbsp	101	10	2	3	1
Almond butter, w/o salt	1 tbsp	101	10	2	3	1
Almonds, roasted	1 oz. (12 nuts)	169	15	6	6	3
Anchovies	3 oz.	111	4	17	0	0
Apple cider, powdered	1 packet	83	0	0	21	0
Apple juice	8 fl.oz.	120	0	0	29	0
Apples, w/o skin	1 medium	61	0	0	16	2
Apples, w/ skin	1 medium	72	0	0	19	3
Applesauce	1 cup	194	1	1	51	3
Apricots	1 apricot	17	0	1	4	1
Arrowroot	1 cup, sliced	78	0	5	16	2
Arrowroot flour	1 cup	457	0	0	113	4
Artichokes	1 artichoke	76	0	5	17	9
Arugula	1 cup	4	0	1	1	0
Asparagus	1 spear	2	0	0	1	0
Avocados	1 cup, cubes	240	22	3	13	10
B						
Bacon bits, meatless	1 tbsp	33	2	2	2	1
Bacon, Canadian, cooked	1 slice	43	2	6	0	0
Bacon, meatless	1 slice	16	2	1	0	0
Bacon, pork, cooked	1 slice	42	3	3	0	0
Bagels, cinnamon-raisin	1 bagel, 4" dia	244	2	9	49	2
Bagels, egg	1 bagel, 4" dia	292	2	11	56	2
Bagels, oat-bran	1 bagel, 4" dia	227	1	10	47	3
Bagels, plain	1 bagel, 4" dia	245	1	9	47	2
Bagels, deli gourmet style	1 bagel	370	3	13	71	2
Balsam pear	1 balsam pear	21	0	1	5	4
Bamboo shoots	1 cup	41	1	4	8	3
Banana chips	1 oz.	147	10	1	17	2

Nutrition values for fat, protein (Prtn), carbohydrates (Cbs), and fiber (Fbr)
are listed in grams per serving. Serving sizes and values are approximate.

FOOD ITEM	Serving Size	Cal	Fat	Prtn	Cbs	Fbr
B (cont.)						
Bananas	1 medium, 7"-8"	105	0	1	27	3
Barley	1 cup	651	4	23	135	32
Barley flour	1 cup	511	2	16	110	15
Barley, pearled, cooked	1 cup	193	1	4	44	6
Basil	5 leaves	1	0	0	0	0
Basil, dried	1 tsp	2	0	0	0	0
Bay leaf	1 tsp, crumbled	2	0	0	0	0
Beans, adzuki, cooked	1 cup	294	0	17	57	17
Beans, baked, canned, plain	1 cup	239	1	12	54	10
Beans, baked, canned, no salt	1 cup	266	1	12	52	13
Beans, baked, canned, w/ beef	1 cup	322	9	17	45	10
Beans, black, cooked	1 cup	227	1	15	40	15
Beans, cranberry, cooked	1 cup	241	1	16	43	18
Beans, fava, canned	1 cup	182	1	14	31	10
Beans, french, cooked	1 cup	228	1	12	43	17
Beans, great northern, cooked	1 cup	209	1	15	37	12
Beans, kidney, cooked	1 cup	225	1	15	40	11
Beans, lima, cooked	1 cup	216	1	15	39	13
Beans, lima, canned	1 can	190	0	12	36	11
Beans, mung, cooked	1 cup	212	1	14	39	15
Beans, mungo, cooked	1 cup	189	1	14	33	12
Beans, navy, cooked	1 cup	255	1	15	47	19
Beans, pink, cooked	1 cup	252	1	15	47	9
Beans, pinto, cooked	1 cup	245	1	15	44	15
Beans, small white, cooked	1 cup	254	1	16	46	18
Beans, snap, green, cooked	1 cup	44	0	2	10	4
Beans, snap, yellow, cooked	1 cup	44	0	2	10	4
Beans, white, cooked	1 cup	249	1	17	45	11
Beans, yellow	1 cup	255	2	16	48	18
Beechnuts, dried	1 oz.	163	14	2	10	0
Beef, choice short rib, cooked	3 oz.	400	36	18	0	0
Beef bologna	1 slice	88	8	3	1	0
Beef jerky, chopped	1 piece	81	5	7	2	0
Beef sausage, precooked	1 link	134	12	6	1	0
Beef stew, canned	1 serving	218	13	12	16	4
Beef, tri-tip roast, roasted	3 oz.	174	9	22	0	0
Beef, brisket, lean & fat, roasted	3 oz.	328	27	20	0	0
Beef, brisket, lean, roasted	3 oz.	206	11	25	0	0
Beef, chuck, arm roast, lean & fat, braised	3 oz.	283	20	23	0	0
Beef, chuck, arm roast, lean, braised	3 oz.	179	7	28	0	0

Nutrition values for fat, protein (Prtn), carbohydrates (Cbs), and fiber (Fbr)
are listed in grams per serving. Serving sizes and values are approximate.

FOOD ITEM	Serving Size	Cal	Fat	Prtn	Cbs	Fbr
B (cont.)						
Beef, chuck, top blade, raw	3 oz.	138	8	17	0	0
Beef, cured breakfast strips	3 slices	276	26	9	1	0
Beef, cured, corned, canned	3 oz.	213	13	23	0	0
Beef, cured, dried	1 serving	43	1	9	1	0
Beef, cured, luncheon meat	1 slice	31	1	5	0	0
Beef, flank, raw	1 oz.	47	2	6	0	0
Beef, ground patties, frozen	3 oz.	240	20	15	0	0
Beef, ground, 70% lean, raw	1 oz.	94	9	4	0	0
Beef, ground, 80% lean, raw	1 oz.	72	6	5	0	0
Beef, ground, 95% lean, raw	1 oz.	39	1	6	0	0
Beef, rib, large end, boneless, raw	1 oz.	94	8	5	0	0
Beef, rib, shortribs, boneless, raw	1 oz.	110	10	4	0	0
Beef, rib, whole, boneless, raw	1 oz.	91	8	5	0	0
Beef, rib-eye, small end, raw	1 oz.	78	6	5	0	0
Beef, round, bottom, raw	1 oz.	56	3	6	0	0
Beef, round, eye, raw	1 oz.	49	3	6	0	0
Beef, round, full cut, raw	1 oz.	55	3	6	0	0
Beef, round, tip, raw	1 oz.	56	4	6	0	0
Beef, round, top, raw	1 oz.	48	2	6	0	0
Beef, shank crosscuts, raw	1 oz.	50	3	6	0	0
Beef, short loin, porterhouse, raw	1 oz.	73	6	5	0	0
Beef, short loin, t-bone, raw	1 oz.	66	5	5	0	0
Beef, short loin, top, raw	1 oz.	66	5	6	0	0
Beef, sirloin, tri-tip, raw	1 oz.	50	3	6	0	0
Beef, tenderloin, raw	1 oz.	70	5	6	0	0
Beef, top sirloin, raw	1 oz.	61	4	6	0	0
Beer, light	12 fl.oz.	110	12	5	7	0
Beer, nonalcoholic	12 fl.oz.	80	1	0	70	0
Beer, regular	12 fl.oz.	140	12	1	10	1
Beets	1 beet	35	0	2	8	4
Bratwurst, chicken	1 serving	148	9	16	0	0
Bratwurst, pork	1 serving	281	25	12	2	0
Bratwurst, veal	1 serving	286	27	12	0	0
Bread stuffing, dry mix, prepared	1/2 cup	178	9	3	22	3
Bread, banana	1 slice	196	6	3	33	1
Bread, corn	1 piece	188	6	4	29	1
Bread, cracked-wheat	1 slice	65	1	2	12	1
Bread, french	1 slice	70	1	3	15	1
Bread, garlic	1 slice	160	10	3	14	1
Bread, Irish soda	1 oz.	82	1	2	16	1

Nutrition values for fat, protein (Prtn), carbohydrates (Cbs), and fiber (Fbr)
are listed in grams per serving. Serving sizes and values are approximate.

FOOD ITEM	Serving Size	Cal	Fat	Prtn	Cbs	Fbr
B (cont.)						
Bread, pita	2 oz.	150	1	3	30	0
Bread, pumpernickel	1 slice	75	1	3	15	2
Bread, raisin	1 slice	80	2	2	15	1
Bread, rice bran	1 oz.	69	1	3	12	1
Bread, sandwich slice	1 slice	70	1	2	13	1
Bread, sourdough	1 slice	100	1	2	20	1
Broad beans, cooked	1 cup	187	1	13	33	9
Brownies	1 brownie	220	13	1	27	1
Buckwheat	1 cup	583	6	23	122	17
Buckwheat flour	1 cup	402	4	15	85	12
Buckwheat groats, roasted, cooked	1 cup	155	1	6	34	5
Buffalo, raw	1 oz.	28	0	6	0	0
Burbot, raw	3 oz.	77	1	16	0	0
Burdock root	1 cup	85	0	2	21	4
Butter, whipped, w/ salt	1 tbsp	67	8	0	0	0
Butternuts, dried	1 oz.	174	16	7	3	1
C						
Cabbage, common	1 cup, shredded	17	1	1	4	2
Cabbage, pak choi	1 cup, shredded	9	0	1	2	1
Cabbage, pe-tsai	1 cup, shredded	12	0	1	3	1
Cake, angel food	1 slice	180	4	2	36	2
Cake, Boston cream pie	1 slice	260	9	1	32	0
Cake, carrot	1 slice	310	16	1	39	0
Cake, cheesecake	1 slice	500	30	4	50	0
Cake, chocolate	1 slice	270	13	1	36	1
Cake, chocolate mousse	1 slice	250	10	1	35	1
Cake, devil's food	1 slice	270	13	2	35	0
Cake, pineapple upside-down	1 piece	367	14	4	58	1
Cake, pound	1 slice	320	16	2	38	0
Cake, sponge cake w/ cream, berries	1 slice	325	8	25	38	1
Cake, yellow	1 slice	260	11	2	36	1
Candy, butterscotch	5 pieces	120	3	0	20	0
Candy, caramels	1 piece	30	1	3	6	1
Candy, carob	1 bar	470	27	7	49	3
Candy, chocolate fudge	1 oz.	125	5	0	18	0
Candy, chocolate mints	1 mint	45	1	0	9	0
Candy, milk chocolate w/ almonds	2 oz.	216	14	4	21	3
Candy, chocolate-coated peanut butter bites	1 piece	45	3	1	4	0
Candy, chocolate-coated peanuts	12 peanuts	160	11	20	15	7

Nutrition values for fat, protein (Prtn), carbohydrates (Cbs), and fiber (Fbr)
are listed in grams per serving. Serving sizes and values are approximate.

NUTRITION FACTS

FOOD ITEM	Serving Size	Cal	Fat	Prtn	Cbs	Fbr
C (cont.)						
Candy, gumdrops	4 pieces	130	0	0	31	0
Candy, hard candy	1 piece	18	0	0	5	0
Candy, jelly beans	12 beans	100	0	0	24	0
Candy, licorice	1 piece	30	0	0	7	0
Candy, lollipop	1 lollipop	20	0	0	5	0
Candy, milk chocolate bar	2 oz.	235	13	3	26	2
Candy, mints	1 mint	30	0	0	7	0
Cantaloupe	1 cup, cubed	54	0	1	13	1
Cardoon	1 cup, shredded	36	0	1	9	3
Carrots	1 medium	65	0	1	15	4
Cashew butter, w/ salt	1 tbsp	94	8	3	4	0
Cashew nuts	1 oz.	157	12	5	9	1
Cassava	1 cup	330	1	3	78	4
Celeraic	1 cup	66	1	2	14	3
Chard, swiss	1 cup	7	0	1	1	1
Cheese, American	1 slice	110	9	5	1	0
Cheese, brick	1 oz.	100	8	31	0	0
Cheese, brie	1 oz.	95	8	50	1	0
Cheese, camembert	1 oz.	90	7	49	1	0
Cheese, cheddar	1 oz.	110	9	33	1	0
Cheese, colby jack	1 oz.	110	9	31	1	0
Cheese, cottage, 2%	1 cup	203	4	31	8	0
Cheese, edam	1 oz.	100	8	7	0	0
Cheese, feta	1 oz.	100	8	21	1	0
Cheese, goat	1 oz.	128	10	9	1	0
Cheese, goat, semisoft	1 oz.	103	9	6	1	0
Cheese, goat, soft	1 oz.	76	6	5	0	0
Cheese, gouda	1 oz.	100	8	7	1	0
Cheese, monterey jack	1 oz.	110	9	32	0	0
Cheese, mozzarella	1 oz.	90	7	25	1	0
Cheese, parmesan, hard	1 oz.	110	7	10	1	0
Cheese, parmesan, shredded	1 tbsp	22	2	2	0	0
Cheese, provolone	1 oz.	100	8	34	1	0
Cheese, queso	2 tbsp	110	9	28	2	0
Cheese, ricotta	2 tbsp	50	4	28	1	0
Cheese, roquefort	1 oz.	105	9	6	1	0
Cheese, swiss	1 oz.	110	9	36	1	0
Cherries, sour	8 pieces	30	0	1	7	2
Cherries, sweet	8 pieces	30	0	2	7	2
Chewing gum	1 piece	25	0	0	5	0

Nutrition values for fat, protein (Prtn), carbohydrates (Cbs), and fiber (Fbr)
are listed in grams per serving. Serving sizes and values are approximate.

FOOD ITEM	Serving Size	Cal	Fat	Prtn	Cbs	Fbr
C (cont.)						
Chicken, breast, w/ skin	1/2 breast	249	13	30	0	0
Chicken, breast, w/o skin	1/2 breast	130	2	27	0	0
Chicken, capons, boneless	1/2 capon	1459	74	184	0	0
Chicken, capons, giblets, cooked	1 cup	238	8	38	1	0
Chicken, cornish game hen, roasted	1/2 bird	336	24	29	0	0
Chicken, cornish game hen, meat only	1 bird	295	9	51	0	0
Chicken, dark meat, w/o skin	1 cup diced	287	14	38	0	0
Chicken, drumstick, w/ skin	1 drumstick	118	6	14	0	0
Chicken, drumstick, w/o skin	1 drumstick	74	2	13	0	0
Chicken, leg, w/ skin	1 leg	312	20	30	0	0
Chicken, leg, w/o skin	1 leg	156	5	26	0	0
Chicken, light meat, w/o skin	1 cup diced	214	6	38	0	0
Chicken, thigh, w/ skin	1 thigh	198	14	16	0	0
Chicken, thigh, w/o skin	1 thigh	82	3	14	0	0
Chicken, wing, w/ skin	1 wing	109	8	9	0	0
Chicken, wing, w/o skin	1 wing	37	1	6	0	0
Chickpeas, cooked	1 cup	269	4	15	45	13
Chicory greens	1 cup, chopped	41	1	3	9	7
Chicory roots	1/2 cup	33	0	1	8	0
Chicory, witloof	1/2 cup	8	0	0	2	1
Chili con carne w/ beans	1 cup	298	13	18	28	10
Chili powder	1 tsp	8	0	0	1	1
Chili w/ beans, canned	1 cup	287	14	15	31	11
Chili w/o beans, canned	1 cup	194	7	17	18	3
Chinese chestnuts	1 oz.	64	0	1	14	0
Chives	1 tbsp, chopped	1	0	0	0	0
Chocolate chip crisped rice bar	1 bar	115	4	1	21	1
Chocolate chips	1/4 cup	210	12	3	24	1
Chocolate milkshake, ready-to-drink	8 fl.oz.	181	5	8	26	1
Chocolate, semi sweet bars, baking	1 oz.	160	8	3	20	1
Chocolate, unsweetened baking squares	1 square	144	15	4	9	5
Chorizo, pork and beef	1 link	273	23	15	1	0
Chow mein noodles	1 cup	237	14	4	26	2
Cinnamon, ground	1 tsp	6	0	0	2	1
Cisco	3 oz.	83	2	16	0	0
Citrus fruit drink, from concentrate	8 fl.oz.	124	0	1	30	1
Clam, mixed species, raw	1 large	15	0	3	1	0
Cloves, ground	1 tsp	7	0	0	1	1
Cocktail mix, nonalcoholic	1 fl.oz.	103	0	0	26	0
Cocoa mix, powder	1 serving	113	1	2	24	1

Nutrition values for fat, protein (Prtn), carbohydrates (Cbs), and fiber (Fbr)
are listed in grams per serving. Serving sizes and values are approximate.

FOOD ITEM	Serving Size	Cal	Fat	Prtn	Cbs	Fbr
C (cont.)						
Cocoa mix, powder, unsweetened	1 tbsp	12	1	1	3	2
Coconut meat	1 cup, shredded	283	27	3	12	7
Coconut milk	1 cup	552	57	6	13	5
Coffee, brewed, decaf	1 cup	0	0	0	0	0
Coffee, brewed, regular	1 cup	2	0	0	0	0
Coffee, café au lait	8 fl.oz.	65	3	1	6	0
Coffee, cappuccino	8 fl.oz.	70	4	1	6	0
Coffee, espresso	1 shot	4	0	0	1	0
Coffee, instant, decaf	1 tsp	0	0	0	0	0
Coffee, instant, regular	1 tsp, dry	2	0	0	0	0
Coffee, latte	8 fl.oz.	100	5	0	8	0
Coffee, mocha	8 fl.oz.	180	12	1	16	0
Coffeecake	3 oz.	230	7	4	38	4
Coleslaw	1/2 cup	41	2	1	7	1
Collards	1 cup, chopped	11	0	1	2	1
Conch, baked or broiled	1 cup, sliced	165	2	33	2	0
Cookies, animal crackers	1 cookie	22	1	0	4	0
Cookies, brownies	4 oz.	430	25	1	52	1
Cookies, butter	1 cookie	23	1	0	3	0
Cookies, chocolate chip, deli fresh baked	1 cookie	275	15	0	38	1
Cookies, chocolate chip, commercial	1 cookie	130	7	1	17	1
Cookies, chocolate chip, refrigerated dough	1 portion	128	6	1	18	0
Cookies, chocolate wafers	1 wafer	26	1	0	4	0
Cookies, fig bars	1 cookie	150	3	2	31	2
Cookies, fudge	1 cookie	73	1	1	16	1
Cookies, gingersnap	1 cookie	29	1	0	5	0
Cookies, graham, plain or honey	2 1/2" square	30	1	1	5	0
Cookies, marshmallow w/ chocolate coating	1 cookie	118	5	1	19	1
Cookies, molasses	1 cookie	138	4	2	24	0
Cookies, oatmeal	1 cookie	238	9	3	38	2
Cookies, oatmeal w/ raisins	1 cookie	238	9	3	38	2
Cookies, oatmeal, commercial, iced	1 cookie	123	5	1	18	1
Cookies, oatmeal, refrigerated dough	1 portion	68	3	1	10	0
Cookies, peanut butter sandwich	1 cookie	67	3	1	9	0
Cookies, peanut butter, refrigerated dough	1 portion	73	4	1	8	0
Cookies, sugar	1 cookie	66	3	1	8	0
Cookies, sugar wafers w/ cream filling	1 wafer	46	2	0	6	0
Cookies, sugar, refrigerated dough	1 portion	113	5	1	15	0
Cookies, vanilla wafers	1 wafer	28	1	0	4	0
Coriander leaves	9 sprigs	5	0	0	1	1

Nutrition values for fat, protein (Prtn), carbohydrates (Cbs), and fiber (Fbr)
are listed in grams per serving. Serving sizes and values are approximate.

FOOD ITEM	Serving Size	Cal	Fat	Prtn	Cbs	Fbr
C (cont.)						
Corn flour, yellow	1 cup	416	4	11	87	0
Corn, sweet, white	1 ear	77	1	3	17	2
Corn, sweet, yellow	1 ear	77	1	3	17	2
Corn, sweet, white, cream style	1 cup	184	1	5	46	3
Corn, sweet, yellow, cream style	1 cup	184	1	5	46	3
Cornnuts	1 oz.	126	4	2	20	2
Cornstarch	1 cup	488	0	0	117	1
Couscous, cooked	1 cup	176	0	6	37	0
Cowpeas (black-eyed peas), cooked	1 cup	160	1	5	34	8
Cowpeas, catjang, cooked	1 cup	200	1	14	35	6
Cowpeas, leafy tips	1 cup, chopped	10	0	2	2	0
Crab, Alaska king, raw	1 leg	144	1	32	0	0
Crab, blue, canned	1 cup	134	2	28	0	0
Crab, dungeness, cooked	1 crab	140	2	28	1	0
Crabapples	1 cup, sliced	84	0	0	22	0
Crackers w/ cheese filling	6 crackers	191	10	4	23	1
Crackers w/ peanut butter filling	6 cracker	193	10	5	22	1
Crackers, cheese, regular	6 crackers	312	16	6	36	2
Crackers, graham	1 cracker	30	1	6	5	2
Crackers, matzo, plain	1 matzo	112	0	3	24	1
Crackers, matzo, whole-wheat	1 matzo	100	0	4	22	3
Crackers, melba toast	1 cup	129	1	4	25	2
Crackers, milk	1 cracker	50	2	1	8	0
Crackers, regular	1 cup, bite size	311	16	5	38	1
Crackers, rusk toast	1 rusk	41	1	1	7	0
Crackers, rye	1 cracker	37	0	1	9	3
Crackers, saltines	1 cracker	20	0	1	4	0
Crackers, soda	1 cracker	60	2	6	10	2
Crackers, wheat	1 cracker	9	0	0	1	0
Crackers, wheat, sandwich w/ peanut butter	1 cracker	35	2	1	4	0
Crackers, whole-wheat	1 cracker	18	1	0	3	0
Cranberries	1 cup, whole	44	0	0	12	4
Cranberry juice cocktail	1 cup	144	0	0	36	0
Cranberry-apple juice	1 cup	174	0	0	44	0
Cranberry-grape juice	1 cup	137	0	1	34	0
Crayfish, wild, raw	8 crayfish	21	0	4	0	0
Cream cheese	1 tbsp	51	5	1	0	0
Cream of tartar	1 tsp	8	0	0	2	0
Cream, half & half	1 tbsp	20	2	0	1	0
Cream, heavy whipping	1 cup, fluid	821	88	5	7	0

Nutrition values for fat, protein (Prtn), carbohydrates (Cbs), and fiber (Fbr) are listed in grams per serving. Serving sizes and values are approximate.

FOOD ITEM	Serving Size	Cal	Fat	Prtn	Cbs	Fbr
C (cont.)						
Crepes	1 crepe	120	6	2	14	1
Croissants, apple	1 croissant	145	5	4	21	1
Croissants, butter	1 croissant	115	6	2	13	1
Croissants, cheese	1 croissant	174	9	4	20	1
Croutons, plain	1 cup	122	2	4	22	2
Croutons, seasoned	1 cup	186	7	4	25	2
Cucumber	1 cucumber	45	0	2	11	2
Cucumber, peeled	1 cup, sliced	14	0	1	3	1
Cumin seed	1 tsp	8	1	0	1	0
Currants, black	1 cup	71	1	2	17	0
Currants, red & white	1 cup	63	0	2	16	5
Curry powder	1 tsp	7	0	0	1	1
D						
Dandelion greens	1 cup, chopped	25	0	2	5	2
Danish pastry, cheese, 4 1/4" diameter	1 pastry	266	16	6	26	1
Danish pastry, cinnamon, 4 1/4" diameter	1 pastry	262	15	5	29	1
Danish pastry, fruit, 4 1/4" diameter	1 pastry	263	13	4	34	1
Danish pastry, nut, 4 1/4" diameter	1 pastry	280	16	5	30	1
Danish pastry, raspberry, 4 1/4" diameter	1 pastry	263	13	4	34	1
Deer, ground, raw	1 oz.	45	2	6	0	0
Deer, raw	1 oz.	34	1	7	0	0
Doughnuts, chocolate coated or frosted	1 doughnut	133	9	1	13	1
Doughnuts, chocolate, sugared or glazed	1 doughnut	250	12	3	34	1
Doughnuts, french crullers	1 cruller	169	8	1	24	1
Doughnuts, plain	1 doughnut, stick	219	12	3	26	1
Doughnuts, wheat, sugared or glazed	1 doughnut	101	5	2	12	1
Duck liver, raw	1 liver	60	2	8	2	0
Duck, meat only, roasted	1/2 duck	444	25	52	0	0
Duck, white pekin, breast w/skin, roasted	1/2 breast	242	13	29	0	0
Duck, skinless, raw	1/2 duck	400	18	55	0	0
Durian	1 cup, chopped	357	13	4	66	9
E						
Eclairs w/ chocolate glaze	1 éclair	293	18	7	27	1
Eel, mixed species, raw	3 oz.	156	10	16	0	0
Egg noodles, cooked	1 cup	213	2	8	40	2
Egg substitute, liquid	1 tbsp	13	1	2	0	0
Egg white, fried	1 large	92	7	6	0	0
Egg white, raw	1 large	17	0	4	0	0

Nutrition values for fat, protein (Prtn), carbohydrates (Cbs), and fiber (Fbr) are listed in grams per serving. Serving sizes and values are approximate.

FOOD ITEM	Serving Size	Cal	Fat	Prtn	Cbs	Fbr
E (cont.)						
Egg yolk, raw	1 large	53	4	3	1	0
Egg, hard-boiled	1 cup, chopped	211	14	17	2	0
Egg, omelette	1 large	93	7	7	0	0
Egg, poached	1 large	74	5	6	0	0
Egg, raw	1 large	85	5.8	7	0	0
Egg, scrambled	1 cup	365	27	24	5	0
Eggnog	8 fl.oz.	343	19	10	34	0
Eggplant	1 eggplant	110	10	5	26	16
Elderberries	1 cup	106	1	1	27	10
Elk, ground, raw	1 oz.	49	3	6	0	0
Elk, raw	1 oz.	31	0	7	0	0
Endive	1 head	87	1	6	17	16
English muffins, plain	1 muffin	134	1	4	26	2
English muffins, cinnamon-raisin	1 muffin	139	2	4	49	2
English muffins, wheat	1 muffin	127	1	5	26	3
English muffins, whole-wheat	1 muffin	134	1	6	27	4
English muffins, whole-wheat/multigrain	1 muffin	155	1	6	31	2
European chestnuts, peeled	1 oz.	56	0	1	13	0
European chestnuts, unpeeled	1 oz.	60	1	1	13	2
F						
Farina, cooked	1 cup.	471	0	3	24	1
Fast food, biscuit w/ egg	1 biscuit	373	22	12	32	1
Fast food, biscuit w/ egg & bacon	1 biscuit	458	31	17	29	1
Fast food, biscuit w/ egg, bacon & cheese	1 biscuit	477	31	16	33	0
Fast food, biscuit w/ sausage	1 biscuit	485	32	12	40	1
Fast food, caramel sundae	1 sundae	304	9	7	49	0
Fast food, cheeseburger, large, double patty	1 sandwich	704	44	38	40	1
Fast food, cheeseburger, large, single patty	1 sandwich	563	33	28	38	1
Fast food, corndog	1 corndog	460	19	17	56	1
Fast food, croissant w/ egg, cheese	1 croissant	368	25	13	24	1
Fast food, croissant w/ egg, cheese, bacon	1 croissant	413	28	16	24	1
Fast food, croissant w/ egg, cheese, sausage	1 croissant	523	38	20	25	1
Fast food, Danish pastry, cheese	1 pastry	353	25	6	29	2
Fast food, Danish pastry, cinnamon	1 pastry	349	17	5	47	2
Fast food, Danish pastry, fruit	1 pastry	335	16	5	45	2
Fast food, fish sandwich w/ tartar sauce	1 sandwich	431	23	17	41	1
Fast food, french toast sticks	5 pieces	513	29	8	58	3
Fast food, fried chicken, boneless	6 pieces	285	18	15	16	1
Fast food, hamburger, large, double patty	1 sandwich	540	27	34	40	2

Nutrition values for fat, protein (Prtn), carbohydrates (Cbs), and fiber (Fbr) are listed in grams per serving. Serving sizes and values are approximate.

NUTRITION FACTS

F (cont.)

FOOD ITEM	Serving Size	Cal	Fat	Prtn	Cbs	Fbr
Fast food, hamburger, large, single patty	1 sandwich	425	21	23	37	2
Fast food, hot fudge sundae	1 sundae	284	9	6	48	0
Fast food, hot dog w/ chili	1 hot dog	296	13	14	31	1
Fast food, hot dog, plain	1 hot dog	242	15	10	18	1
Fast food, McDonald's Big Mac® w/ cheese	1 serving	560	30	25	46	3
Fast food, McDonald's Big Mac® w/o cheese	1 serving	495	25	23	43	3
Fast food, McDonald's cheeseburger	1 serving	310	12	15	35	1
Fast food, McDonald's Chicken McGrill®	1 serving	400	16	27	38	3
Fast food, McDonald's Crispy Chicken	1 serving	500	23	24	50	3
Fast food, McDonald's Filet-o-Fish®	1 serving	400	18	14	42	1
Fast food, McDonald's french fries	1 medium	350	11	4	47	5
Fast food, McDonald's hamburger	1 serving	260	9	13	33	1
Fast food, McDonald's 1/4 Pounder®,cheese	1 serving	510	25	29	43	3
Fast food, McDonald's 1/4 Pounder®	1 serving	420	18	24	40	3
Fast food, onion rings, 8-9 rings	1 portion	276	16	4	31	3
Fast food, strawberry sundae	1 sundae	268	8	6	45	0
Fast food, submarine sandwich w/ cold cuts	1 submarine 6"	456	19	22	51	4
Fast food, submarine sandwich w/ roast beef	1 submarine 6"	410	13	29	44	4
Fast food, submarine sandwich w/ tuna	1 submarine 6"	584	28	30	55	4
Fast food, vanilla soft-serve w/ cone	1 cone	164	6	4	24	0
Fennel bulb	1 cup, sliced	27	0	1	6	3
Fennel seed	1 tbsp	20	1	1	3	2
Fenugreek seed	1 tbsp	36	1	3	7	3
Figs	1 medium	37	0	0	10	2
Figs, dried	1 fig	21	0	0	5	1
Fireweed leaves	1 cup, chopped	24	1	1	4	2
Fish oil, cod liver	1 tbsp	123	14	0	0	0
Fish oil, herring	1 tbsp	123	14	0	0	0
Fish oil, menhaden	1 tbsp	123	14	0	0	0
Fish oil, salmon	1 tbsp	123	14	0	0	0
Fish oil, sardine	1 tbsp	123	14	0	0	0
Fish, bluefin tuna, raw	3 oz.	122	4	20	0	0
Fish, bluefish, raw	3 oz.	105	4	17	0	0
Fish, butterfish, raw	3 oz.	124	7	15	0	0
Fish, carp, raw	3 oz.	108	5	15	0	0
Fish, catfish, raw	3 oz.	81	2	14	0	0
Fish, cod, Atlantic, raw	3 oz.	70	1	15	0	0
Fish, croaker, Atlantic, raw	3 oz.	88	3	15	0	0
Fish, flatfish, raw	3 oz.	77	1	16	0	0
Fish, gefilte fish	1 piece	35	1	4	3	0

Nutrition values for fat, protein (Prtn), carbohydrates (Cbs), and fiber (Fbr) are listed in grams per serving. Serving sizes and values are approximate.

FOOD ITEM	Serving Size	Cal	Fat	Prtn	Cbs	Fbr
F (cont.)						
Fish, grouper, mixed species, raw	3 oz.	78	1	17	0	0
Fish, haddock, raw	3 oz.	74	1	16	0	0
Fish, halibut, raw	3 oz.	94	2	18	0	0
Fish, herring, Atlantic, raw	3 oz.	134	8	15	0	0
Fish, herring, pacific, raw	3 oz.	166	12	14	0	0
Fish, mackerel, Atlantic, raw	3 oz.	174	12	16	0	0
Fish, mackerel, king, raw	3 oz.	89	2	17	0	0
Fish, mackerel, pacific, raw	3 oz.	134	7	17	0	0
Fish, mackerel, Spanish, raw	3 oz.	118	5	16	0	0
Fish, milkfish, raw	3 oz.	126	6	18	0	0
Fish, monkfish, raw	3 oz.	65	1	12	0	0
Fish, ocean perch, Atlantic, raw	3 oz.	80	1	16	0	0
Fish, perch, mixed species, raw	3 oz.	77	1	17	0	0
Fish, pike, northern, raw	3 oz.	75	1	16	0	0
Fish, pollock, Atlantic, raw	3 oz.	78	1	17	0	0
Fish, pout, ocean, raw	3 oz.	67	1	14	0	0
Fish, rainbow smelt, raw	3 oz.	82	2	15	0	0
Fish, rockfish, pacific, raw	3 oz.	80	1	16	0	0
Fish, roe, mixed species, raw	1 tbsp	20	10	3	0	0
Fish, sablefish, raw	3 oz.	166	13	11	0	0
Fish, salmon, Atlantic, farmed, raw	3 oz.	156	9	17	0	0
Fish, salmon, Atlantic, wild, raw	3 oz.	121	5	17	0	0
Fish, salmon, chinook, raw	3 oz.	152	9	17	0	0
Fish, salmon, pink, raw	3 oz.	99	3	17	0	0
Fish, sea bass, mixed species, raw	3 oz.	82	2	16	0	0
Fish, seatrout, mixed species, raw	3 oz.	88	3	14	0	0
Fish, shad, raw	3 oz.	167	12	14	0	0
Fish, skipjack tuna, raw	3 oz.	88	1	19	0	0
Fish, snapper, mixed species, raw	3 oz.	85	1	17	0	0
Fish, striped bass, raw	3 oz.	82	2	15	0	0
Fish, striped mullet	3 oz.	99	3	16	0	0
Fish, sturgeon, mixed species, raw	3 oz.	89	3	14	0	0
Fish, swordfish, raw	3 oz.	103	3	17	0	0
Fish, trout, mixed species, raw	3 oz.	126	6	18	0	0
Fish, white sucker, raw	3 oz.	78	2	14	0	0
Fish, whitefish, raw	3 oz.	114	5	16	0	0
Fish, wolffish, Atlantic, raw	3 oz.	82	2	15	0	0
Fish, yellowfin tuna, raw	3 oz.	93	1	20	0	0
Fish, yellowtail, mixed species, raw	3 oz.	124	5	20	0	0
Flan, caramel custard	5 1/2 oz.	303	12	4	43	0

Nutrition values for fat, protein (Prtn), carbohydrates (Cbs), and fiber (Fbr) are listed in grams per serving. Serving sizes and values are approximate.

FOOD ITEM	Serving Size	Cal	Fat	Prtn	Cbs	Fbr
F (cont.)						
Flaxseed	1 tbsp	59	4	2	4	3
Flaxseed oil	1 tbsp	120	14	0	0	0
Frankfurter	1 serving	151	13	5	2	0
Frankfurter, beef	1 frankfurter	188	17	6	2	0
Frankfurter, beef & pork	1 frankfurter	174	16	7	1	1
Frankfurter, chicken	1 frankfurter	116	9	6	3	0
Frankfurter, meat	1 frankfurter	151	13	5	2	0
Frankfurter, meatless	1 frankfurter	163	10	14	5	3
Frankfurter, pork	1 frankfurter	204	18	10	0	0
Frankfurter, turkey	1 frankfurter	102	8	6	1	0
French fries, frozen, unprepared, 18 fries	1 serving	170	7	3	28	3
French toast, frozen, ready-to-heat	1 piece	126	4	4	19	1
Frosting, creamy chocolate	2 tbsp	164	7	1	26	0
Frosting, creamy vanilla	2 tbsp	160	6	0	26	0
Frozen yogurt, chocolate, soft-serve	1/2 cup	115	4	3	18	2
Frozen yogurt, vanilla, soft-serve	1/2 cup	117	4	3	17	0
Fruit cocktail, canned	1 cup	229	0	1	60	3
Fruit punch, prepared from concentrate	8 fl.oz.	124	1	0	30	0
Fruit salad, canned in syrup	1 cup	186	0	1	49	3
Fruit salad, canned in water	1 cup	74	0	1	19	3
G						
Garden cress, raw	1 cup	16	0	1	3	1
Garlic	1 clove	4	0	0	1	0
Garlic powder	1 tsp	9	0	1	2	0
Gelatin dessert mix, prepared w/ water	1/2 cup	84	0	2	19	0
Gin, 80 Proof	1 fl.oz.	73	0	0	0	0
Ginger root	1 tsp	2	0	0	0	0
Ginger, ground	1 tsp	6	0	0	1	0
Ginkgo nuts	1 oz.	52	1	1	11	0
Ginkgo nuts, dried	1 oz.	99	1	3	21	0
Goose liver, raw	1 liver	125	4	15	6	0
Goose, meat & skin, roasted	cup chopped	427	31	35	0	0
Goose, meat only, roasted	cup chopped	340	18	41	0	0
Gourd, white-flowered	1 gourd	108	0	5	26	0
Granola bars, hard, plain	1 bar	134	6	3	18	2
Granola bars, soft, plain	1 bar	126	5	2	19	1
Grape juice	8 fl.oz.	160	0	0	40	0
Grapefruit	1/2 fruit	50	0	1	12	3
Grapefruit juice, sweetened	8 fl.oz.	125	0	0	33	0

Nutrition values for fat, protein (Prtn), carbohydrates (Cbs), and fiber (Fbr)
are listed in grams per serving. Serving sizes and values are approximate.

FOOD ITEM	Serving Size	Cal	Fat	Prtn	Cbs	Fbr
G (cont.)						
Grapefruit juice, unsweetened	8 fl.oz.	91	0	1	22	0
Grapes, canned, heavy syrup	1 cup	187	0	1	50	2
Grapes, red or green	1 cup	106	0	1	28	1
Gravy, mushroom, canned	1 can	149	8	4	16	1
Gravy, au jus, canned	1 can	48	1	4	8	0
Gravy, beef, canned	1 can	154	7	11	14	1
Gravy, chicken, canned	1 can	235	17	6	16	1
Gravy, turkey, canned	1 can	152	6	8	15	1
Guacamole dip	2 tbsp	50	4	12	4	0
Guavas	1 fruit	37	1	1	8	3
H						
Ham, chopped	1 slice	50	3	5	1	0
Ham, minced	1 slice	55	4	3	0	0
Ham, sliced	1 slice	46	2	5	1	0
Hazelnuts, dry roasted	1 oz.	183	18	4	5	3
Hazelnuts, blanched	1 oz.	178	17	4	5	3
Hominy, canned, white	1 cup	119	2	2	24	4
Hominy, canned, yellow	1 cup	115	1	2	23	4
Honey	1 tbsp	64	0	0	17	0
Honeydew melons	1 cup, diced	61	0	1	16	1
Horseradish	1 tsp	2	0	0	1	0
Hot chocolate	8 fl.oz.	200	10	9	25	3
Hummus	1 tbsp	23	1	1	2	1
Hush puppies	1 hush puppy	74	3	2	10	1
I						
Ice cream cone, rolled or sugar type	1 cone	40	0	1	8	0
Ice cream cone, wafer or cake type	1 cone	17	0	0	3	0
Ice cream, chocolate	1/2 cup	143	7	3	19	1
Ice cream, strawberry	1/2 cup	127	6	2	18	1
Ice cream, vanilla	1/2 cup	144	8	3	17	1
Iced tea, presweetened	8 fl.oz.	100	0	0	25	0
Iced tea, unsweetened	8 fl.oz.	2	0	0	0	0
Italian seasoning	1 tsp	4	0	0	1	0
J						
Jams and preserves	1 tbsp	56	0	0	14	0
Japanese chestnuts	1 oz.	44	0	1	10	0
Japanese soba noodles, cooked	1 cup	113	0	6	24	2

Nutrition values for fat, protein (Prtn), carbohydrates (Cbs), and fiber (Fbr)
are listed in grams per serving. Serving sizes and values are approximate.

FOOD ITEM	Serving Size	Cal	Fat	Prtn	Cbs	Fbr
J (cont.)						
Japanese ramen noodles, packaged, dry	1 serving	195	7	4	28	1
Jellies	1 tbsp	55	0	0	14	0
K						
Kale	1 cup, chopped	34	1	2	7	1
Kiwifruit	1 medium	45	0	2	11	5
Kumquats	1 fruit	13	0	0	3	1
L						
Lamb, cubed, raw	1 oz.	38	2	6	0	0
Lamb, foreshank, raw	1 oz.	57	4	5	0	0
Lamb, ground, raw	1 oz.	80	7	5	0	0
Lamb, leg, shank half, raw	1 oz.	52	3	5	0	0
Lamb, leg, sirloin half, raw	1 oz.	74	6	5	0	0
Lamb, leg, whole, choice, raw	1 oz.	65	5	5	0	0
Lamb, loin, choice, raw	1 oz.	79	6	5	0	0
Lamb, rib, choice, raw	1 oz.	97	9	4	0	0
Lamb, shoulder, arm, raw	1 oz.	69	5	5	0	0
Lamb, shoulder, blade, raw	1 oz.	69	5	5	0	0
Lamb, shoulder, whole, raw	1 oz.	69	5	5	0	0
Lard	1 tbsp	115	13	0	0	0
Leeks	1 leek	54	0	1	13	2
Lemon juice	1 cup	61	0	1	21	1
Lemon juice, canned or bottled	1 tbsp	3	0	0	1	0
Lemon pepper seasoning	1 tsp	7	0	0	1	0
Lemonade powder	1 scoop	102	0	0	27	0
Lemonade, pink concentrate, prepared	8 fl.oz.	99	0	0	26	0
Lemonade, white concentrate, prepared	8 fl.oz.	131	0	0	34	0
Lemons w/ peel	1 fruit	22	0	1	12	5
Lentils, cooked	1 cup	230	1	18	40	16
Lentils, sprouted, raw	1 cup	82	0	7	17	0
Lettuce, green leaf	1 cup, shredded	5	0	1	1	1
Lettuce, iceberg	1 cup, shredded	10	0	1	2	1
Lettuce, red leaf	1 cup, shredded	3	0	0	0	0
Lettuce, romaine	1 cup, shredded	8	0	1	2	1
Lime juice	1 cup	62	0	1	21	1
Limes	1 fruit	20	0	1	7	2
Liverwurst, pork	1 slice	59	5	3	0	0
Lobster, northern, raw	1 lobster	135	1	28	1	0
Luncheon meat, beef, loaved	1 oz.	87	7	4	1	0

Nutrition values for fat, protein (Prtn), carbohydrates (Cbs), and fiber (Fbr)
are listed in grams per serving. Serving sizes and values are approximate.

FOOD ITEM	Serving Size	Cal	Fat	Prtn	Cbs	Fbr
L (cont.)						
Luncheon meat, beef, thin sliced	1 oz.	50	1	8	2	0
Luncheon meat, meatless slices	1 slice	26	2	3	1	0
Luncheon meat, pork & chicken, minced	1 oz.	56	4	4	0	0
Luncheon meat, pork & ham, minced	1 oz.	88	75	4	1	0
Luncheon meat, pork or beef	1 oz.	99	9	4	1	0
Luncheon meat, pork, canned	1 oz.	95	9	4	1	0
Luncheon meat, pork, ham & chicken, minced	1 oz.	87	8	4	1	0
Luncheon sausage, pork & beef	1 oz.	74	6	4	0	0
M						
Macadamia nuts	1 oz. (10-12 nuts)	203	22	2	4	2
Macaroni and cheese, commercial, prepared	1 cup	259	3	11	48	2
Macaroni, cooked	1 cup	197	1	7	40	2
Malt drink mix, dry	3 heaping tsp	87	2	2	16	0
Malt beverage	8 fl.oz.	144	0	1	32	0
Mangos	1 fruit	135	1	1	35	4
Maraschino cherries	1 cherry	8	0	0	2	0
Margarine, fat free spread	1 tbsp	6	0	0	1	0
Margarine, stick	1 tbsp	100	11	0	0	0
Margarine, stick, unsalted	1 tbsp	102	11	0	0	0
Margarine, tub	1 tbsp	102	11	0	0	0
Martini	1 fl.oz.	69	0	0	1	0
Mayonnaise	1 tbsp	100	11	0	0	0
Milk, 1% low fat	1 cup	102	2	8	12	0
Milk, 2% low fat	1 cup	138	5	10	14	0
Milk, buttermilk, cultured, reduced fat	1 cup	137	5	10	13	0
Milk, chocolate	1 cup	208	9	8	26	2
Milk, dry, nonfat, instant	1/3 cup dry	82	0	8	12	0
Milk, evaporated	1/2 cup	169	10	9	13	0
Milk, skim or nonfat	1 cup	83	0	8	12	0
Milk, canned, sweetened condensed	1 cup	982	27	24	167	0
Milk, whole	1 cup	146	8	8	11	0
Milkshake, dry mix, vanilla	1 envelope packet	69	1	5	11	0
Millet	1 cup	756	8	22	146	17
Miso soup	1 cup	547	17	32	73	15
Mixed nuts	1 cup	814	71	24	35	12
Molasses	1 tablespoon	58	0	0	15	0
Muffins, apple bran	1 muffin	300	3	1	61	1
Muffins, banana nut	1 muffin	480	24	3	60	2
Muffins, blueberry	1 muffin	313	7	6	54	3

Nutrition values for fat, protein (Prtn), carbohydrates (Cbs), and fiber (Fbr)
are listed in grams per serving. Serving sizes and values are approximate.

NUTRITION FACTS

FOOD ITEM	Serving Size	Cal	Fat	Prtn	Cbs	Fbr
M (cont.)						
Muffins, chocolate chip	1 muffin	510	24	2	69	4
Muffins, corn	1 muffin	345	10	7	58	4
Muffins, oat bran	1 muffin	305	8	8	55	5
Muffins, plain	1 muffin	242	9	4	36	2
Mushrooms	1 cup, pieces	15	0	2	2	1
Mushrooms, enoki	1 large	2	0	0	0	0
Mushrooms, oyster	1 large	55	1	6	9	4
Mushrooms, portobello	1 large	0	0	0	0	0
Mushrooms, shiitake	1 mushroom	11	0	0	3	0
Mussels, blue, raw	1 cup	129	3	18	6	0
Mustard greens	1 cup, chopped	15	0	2	3	2
Mustard seed, yellow	1 tbsp	53	3	3	4	2
Mustard spinach	1 cup, chopped	33	1	3	6	4
Mustard, prepared, yellow	1 tsp	3	0	0	0	0
N						
Natto (fermented soybeans)	1 cup	371	19	31	25	10
Nectarines	1 fruit	60	0	1	14	2
New Zealand spinach	1 cup, chopped	8	0	1	1	0
Nutmeg, ground	1 tsp	12	1	0	1	1
O						
Oat bran	1 cup	231	7	16	62	15
Oatmeal, instant, prepared w/ water	1 cup	129	2	5	22	4
Oil, canola	1 tbsp	124	14	0	0	0
Oil, canola & soybean	1 tbsp	119	14	0	0	0
Oil, coconut	1 tbsp	120	14	0	0	0
Oil, corn, peanut & olive	1 tbsp	120	14	0	0	0
Oil, olive	1 tbsp	119	14	0	0	0
Oil, peanut	1 tbsp	119	14	0	0	0
Oil, sesame	1 tbsp	120	14	0	0	0
Oil, soy	1 tbsp	120	14	0	0	0
Oil, vegetable, almond	1 tbsp	120	14	0	0	0
Oil, vegetable, cocoa butter	1 tbsp	120	14	0	0	0
Oil, vegetable, coconut	1 tbsp	117	14	0	0	0
Oil, vegetable, grapeseed	1 tbsp	120	14	0	0	0
Oil, vegetable, hazelnut	1 tbsp	120	14	0	0	0
Oil, vegetable, nutmeg butter	1 tbsp	120	14	0	0	0
Oil, vegetable, palm	1 tbsp	120	14	0	0	0
Oil, vegetable, poppyseed	1 tbsp	120	14	0	0	0

Nutrition values for fat, protein (Prtn), carbohydrates (Cbs), and fiber (Fbr)
are listed in grams per serving. Serving sizes and values are approximate.

FOOD ITEM	Serving Size	Cal	Fat	Prtn	Cbs	Fbr
O (cont.)						
Oil, vegetable, rice bran	1 tbsp	120	14	0	0	0
Oil, vegetable, sheanut	1 tbsp	120	14	0	0	0
Oil, vegetable, tomatoseed	1 tbsp	120	14	0	0	0
Oil, vegetable, walnut	1 tbsp	120	14	0	0	0
Okra	1 cup	31	0	2	7	3
Onion powder	1 tsp	8	0	0	2	0
Onions	1 cup, chopped	67	0	2	16	2
Onions, sweet	1 onion	106	0	3	25	3
Orange juice	8 fl.oz.	109	1	2	25	1
Orange marmalade	1 tbsp	49	0	0	13	0
Oranges	1 large	86	0	2	22	4
Oregano, dried	1 tsp, ground	6	0	0	1	1
Oyster, eastern, raw	3 oz.	50	1	4	5	0
Oyster, pacific, raw	3 oz.	69	2	8	4	0
P						
Pancakes, blueberry	1 pancake	84	4	2	11	0
Pancakes, buttermilk	1 pancake	86	4	3	11	0
Pancakes, plain, dry mix	1 pancake	74	1	2	14	1
Papayas	1 cup, cubed	55	0	1	14	3
Paprika	1 tsp	6	0	0	1	1
Parsley	1 cup	22	1	2	4	2
Parsley, dried	1 tsp	1	0	0	0	0
Parsnips	1 cup, sliced	100	0	2	24	7
Passion fruit	1 fruit	17	0	0	4	2
Pasta, corn, cooked	1 cup	176	1	4	39	7
Pasta, plain, cooked	1 cup	197	1	7	40	2
Pasta, spinach, cooked	1 cup	195	1	8	38	2
Pastrami, turkey	1 oz.	40	2	5	1	0
Pate de foie gras	1 tbsp	60	6	2	1	0
Pate, chicken liver, canned	1 tbsp	26	2	2	1	0
Pate, goose liver, canned	1 tbsp	60	6	2	1	0
Peaches	1 large	61	0	1	15	2
Peaches, canned	1 cup, halved	59	0	1	15	3
Peanut butter, chunky	2 tbsp	188	16	8	7	3
Peanut butter, smooth	2 tbsp	188	16	8	6	2
Peanuts, dry roasted w/ salt	1 oz.	166	14	7	6	2
Peanuts, raw	1 oz.	161	14	7	5	2
Pears	1 pear	121	0	1	32	7
Pears, Asian	1 pear	116	1	1	29	10

Nutrition values for fat, protein (Prtn), carbohydrates (Cbs), and fiber (Fbr)
are listed in grams per serving. Serving sizes and values are approximate.

NUTRITION FACTS

FOOD ITEM	Serving Size	Cal	Fat	Prtn	Cbs	Fbr
P (cont.)						
Pears, canned	1 cup	71	0	1	19	4
Peas, green, fresh, cooked	1 cup	134	0	9	25	9
Peas, green, frozen, cooked	1 cup	125	0	8	23	9
Peas, split, cooked	1 cup	231	1	16	41	16
Pecans	1 oz. (20 halves)	196	20	3	40	3
Pepper, black	1 tsp	5	0	0	1	1
Pepper, red or cayenne	1 tsp	6	0	0	1	1
Pepperoni	15 slices	135	12	6	1	0
Peppers, chili, green	1 cup	29	0	1	6	2
Peppers, chili, red	1 pepper	18	0	1	4	1
Peppers, chili, sun-dried	1 pepper	2	0	0	0	0
Peppers, Jalapeño	1 pepper	4	0	0	1	0
Peppers, sweet, green	1 medium	24	0	1	6	2
Peppers, sweet, red	1 medium	31	0	1	7	2
Peppers, sweet, yellow	1 medium	32	0	1	8	1
Persimmons	1 fruit	32	0	0	8	0
Pheasant, boneless, raw	1/2 pheasant	724	37	91	0	0
Pheasant, breast, skinless, boneless, raw	1/2 breast	242	6	44	0	0
Pheasant, leg, skinless, boneless, raw	1 leg	143	5	24	0	0
Pheasant, skinless, raw	/2 pheasant	468	13	83	0	0
Pickle relish, sweet	1 tbsp	20	0	0	5	0
Pickle, sour	1 large 4"	15	0	0	3	2
Pickle, sweet	1 large 4"	158	0	1	43	2
Pickles, dill	1 large 4"	24	0	1	6	2
Pie crust, graham cracker, baked	1 pie crust	1037	52	9	137	3
Pie, apple	1 piece	411	19	4	58	0
Pie, blueberry	1 piece	290	13	2	44	1
Pie, cherry	1 piece	325	14	3	50	1
Pie, lemon meringue	1 piece	303	10	2	53	1
Pie, pecan	1 piece	452	21	5	65	4
Pie, pumpkin	1 piece	229	10	4	30	3
Pine nuts	1 oz. (167 kernels)	191	19	4	4	1
Pineapple	1 fruit	227	1	3	60	7
Pineapple, canned	1 slice	15	0	0	4	0
Pita bread, whole wheat	1 pita	170	2	6	35	5
Pistachio nuts	1 oz. (49 kernels)	161	13	6	8	3
Pizza, cheese	1 slice (3.7 oz.)	250	10	11	29	2
Pizza, pepperoni	1 slice (3.7 oz.)	288	15	12	26	2
Plantains	1 medium	218	1	2	57	4
Plums	1 fruit	30	0	1	8	1

Nutrition values for fat, protein (Prtn), carbohydrates (Cbs), and fiber (Fbr)
are listed in grams per serving. Serving sizes and values are approximate.

FOOD ITEM	Serving Size	Cal	Fat	Prtn	Cbs	Fbr
P (cont.)						
Plums, canned	1 plum	19	0	0	5	0
Polenta	1/2 cup	220	2	2	24	1
Pomegranates	1 fruit	105	1	2	26	1
Popcorn cakes	1 cake	38	0	1	8	0
Popcorn, air-popped	1 cup	31	0	1	6	1
Popcorn, caramel-coated	1 oz.	122	4	1	22	2
Popcorn, cheese	1 cup	58	4	1	6	1
Popcorn, oil-popped	1 cup	55	3	1	6	1
Popovers, dry mix	1 oz.	105	1	3	20	1
Poppy seed	1 tsp	15	1	1	1	0
Pork, cured, breakfast strips, cooked	3 slices	156	12	10	0	0
Pork, cured, ham, extra lean, canned	3 oz.	116	4	18	0	0
Pork, cured, ham, patties	1 patty	205	18	8	1	0
Pork, cured, ham, extra lean, cooked	3 oz.	140	7	19	0	0
Pork, cured, salt pork, raw	1 oz.	212	23	1	0	0
Pork, fresh ground, cooked	3 oz.	252	18	22	0	0
Pork, leg, rump half, cooked	3 oz.	214	12	25	0	0
Pork, leg, shank half, cooked	3 oz.	246	17	22	0	0
Pork, leg, whole, cooked	3 oz.	232	15	23	0	0
Pork, loin, blade, cooked	3 oz.	275	21	20	0	0
Pork, loin, center loin, cooked	3 oz.	199	11	22	0	0
Pork, loin, center rib, cooked	3 oz.	214	13	23	0	0
Pork, loin, sirloin, cooked	3 oz.	176	8	24	0	0
Pork, loin, tenderloin, cooked	3 oz.	147	5	24	0	0
Pork, loin, top loin, cooked	3 oz.	192	10	24	0	0
Pork, loin, whole, cooked	3 oz.	211	12	23	0	0
Pork, shoulder, arm, cooked	3 oz.	238	18	17	0	0
Pork, shoulder, blade, cooked	3 oz.	229	16	20	0	0
Pork, shoulder, whole, cooked	3 oz.	248	18	20	0	0
Pork, spareribs, cooked	3 oz.	337	26	25	0	0
Potato chips, barbecue	1 oz.	139	9	2	15	1
Potato chips, cheese	1 oz.	141	8	2	16	2
Potato chips, salted	1 oz.	152	10	2	15	1
Potato chips, sour cream & onion	1 oz.	151	10	2	15	2
Potato chips, reduced fat	1 oz.	134	6	2	19	2
Potato chips, unsalted	1 oz.	152	10	2	15	1
Potato flour	1 cup	571	1	11	133	9
Potato salad	1 cup	358	21	7	28	3
Potatoes	1 medium	164	0	4	37	5
Potatoes, baked, w/ skin	1 medium	160	0	4	37	4

Nutrition values for fat, protein (Prtn), carbohydrates (Cbs), and fiber (Fbr)
are listed in grams per serving. Serving sizes and values are approximate.

NUTRITION FACTS

FOOD ITEM	Serving Size	Cal	Fat	Prtn	Cbs	Fbr
P (cont.)						
Potatoes, baked, w/o skin	1 medium	143	0	3	33	3
Potatoes, mashed	1 cup	237	9	4	35	3
Potatoes, red	1 medium	153	0	4	34	4
Potatoes, russet	1 medium	168	0	5	39	3
Potatoes, scalloped	1 cup	211	9	7	26	5
Potatoes, white	1 medium	149	0	4	34	5
Pretzels, hard, plain, salted	1 oz.	108	1	3	22	1
Prune juice	8 fl.oz.	180	0	2	43	3
Pudding, banana	1/2 cup	154	3	4	29	0
Pudding, chocolate	1/2 cup	154	3	5	28	0
Pudding, coconut cream	1/2 cup	157	3	4	28	0
Pudding, lemon	1/2 cup	157	3	4	30	0
Pudding, rice	1/2 cup	163	2	5	31	0
Pudding, tapioca	1/2 cup	154	2	4	29	0
Pudding, vanilla	1/2 cup	148	3	4	27	0
Pumpkin	1 cup	30	0	1	8	1
Pumpkin pie mix	1 cup	281	0	3	71	22
Pumpkin, canned	1 cup	83	1	3	20	7
R						
Rabbit, cooked	3 oz.	167	7	25	0	0
Radicchio	1 cup, shredded	9	0	1	2	0
Radishes	1 cup, sliced	19	0	1	4	2
Raisins	1 1/2 oz.	129	0	1	34	2
Raisins, golden	1 1/2 oz.	130	0	1	34	2
Raspberries	1 cup	64	1	2	15	8
Rhubarb	1 cup, diced	26	0	1	6	2
Rice cakes, brown rice, corn	1 cake	35	0	1	7	0
Rice cakes, brown rice, multigrain	1 cake	35	0	1	7	0
Rice cakes, brown rice, plain	1 cake	35	0	1	7	0
Rice, brown, cooked	1 cup	218	2	5	46	4
Rice, white, cooked	1 cup	242	0	4	53	1
Rice, wild	1 cup	166	1	7	35	3
Rolls, dinner	1 roll	136	3	4	23	1
Rolls, dinner, wheat	1 roll	117	3	4	20	2
Rolls, dinner, whole-wheat	1 roll	114	2	4	22	3
Rolls, french	1 roll	119	2	4	22	0
Rolls, hamburger or hotdog	1 roll	120	2	4	21	1
Rolls, hard (incl. kaiser)	1 roll	126	2	4	23	1
Rolls, pumpernickel	1 roll	119	1	5	23	2

Nutrition values for fat, protein (Prtn), carbohydrates (Cbs), and fiber (Fbr) are listed in grams per serving. Serving sizes and values are approximate.

FOOD ITEM	Serving Size	Cal	Fat	Prtn	Cbs	Fbr
R (cont.)						
Rosemary	1 tsp	1	0	0	0	0
Rosemary, dried	1 tsp	4	0	0	1	1
Rum, 80 proof	1 fl.oz.	64	0	0	0	0
Rutabagas	1 cup, cubed	50	0	2	11	4
Rye	1 cup	566	4	25	118	25
Rye flour, dark	1 cup	415	3	18	88	29
Rye flour, light	1 cup	374	1	9	82	15
Rye flour, medium	1 cup	361	2	10	79	15
S						
Sage, ground	1 tsp	2	0	0	0	0
Sake	1 fl.oz.	39	0	0	2	0
Salad dressing, 1000 island	1 tbsp	58	6	0	2	0
Salad dressing, bacon & tomato	1 tbsp	49	5	0	0	0
Salad dressing, blue cheese	1 tbsp	77	8	1	1	0
Salad dressing, caesar	1 tbsp	78	9	0	1	0
Salad dressing, coleslaw	1 tbsp	61	5	0	4	0
Salad dressing, french	1 tbsp	71	7	0	2	0
Salad dressing, honey dijon	1 tbsp	58	5	1	3	1
Salad dressing, Italian	1 tbsp	43	4	0	2	0
Salad dressing, mayo-based	1 tbsp	57	5	0	4	0
Salad dressing, mayonnaise	1 tbsp	103	12	0	0	0
Salad dressing, peppercorn	1 tbsp	76	8	0	1	0
Salad dressing, ranch	1 tbsp	25	0	0	0	0
Salad dressing, Russian	1 tbsp	76	8	0	2	0
Salad, chicken	6 oz.	420	33	45	11	2
Salad, egg	6 oz.	300	23	20	14	1
Salad, prima pasta	6 oz.	360	30	5	18	3
Salad, seafood w/ crab & shrimp	6 oz.	420	34	0	20	0
Salad, tuna	6 oz.	450	36	16	14	0
Salami, cooked, turkey	1 oz.	38	2	1	0	0
Salami, dry, pork or beef	3 slices	104	8	6	1	0
Salami, Italian pork	1 oz.	119	10	6	0	0
Salsa, w/ oil	2 tbsp	40	3	0	8	0
Salsa, w/o oil	2 tbsp	15	0	0	4	0
Salt	1 tbsp	0	0	0	0	0
Sauce, alfredo	1/4 cup	120	11	15	3	2
Sauce, barbecue	1 cup	188	5	5	32	3
Sauce, cheese	1 cup	479	36	25	13	0
Sauce, cranberry	1 cup	418	0	1	108	3

Nutrition values for fat, protein (Prtn), carbohydrates (Cbs), and fiber (Fbr)
are listed in grams per serving. Serving sizes and values are approximate.

FOOD ITEM	Serving Size	Cal	Fat	Prtn	Cbs	Fbr
S (cont.)						
Sauce, hollandaise	1 cup	62	2	2	10	0
Sauce, honey mustard	1 tbsp	30	1	0	5	0
Sauce, marinara	1 cup	185	6	5	28	1
Sauce, salsa	1 cup	70	0	4	16	4
Sauce, soy	1 tbsp	10	0	0	0	0
Sauce, steak	1 tbsp	25	0	0	6	0
Sauce, teriyaki	1 tbsp	15	0	17	2	0
Sauce, tomato chili	1 cup	284	1	7	54	16
Sauce, worcestershire	1 cup	184	0	0	54	0
Sauerkraut	1/2 cup	25	0	1	5	4
Sausage, Italian pork, raw	1 link	391	35	16	1	0
Sausage, pork	1 link	85	7	4	0	0
Sausage, smoked linked, pork	1 link	265	22	15	1	0
Sausage, turkey	1 link	0	0	0	0	0
Savory, ground	1 tsp	4	0	0	1	1
Scallops	1 scallop	26	0	5	1	0
Seaweed, dried	1 oz.	50	0	0	13	0
Sesame seeds, dried	1 tbsp	52	5	2	2	1
Shallots	1 tbsp, chopped	7	0	0	2	0
Shortening	1 tbsp	113	13	0	0	0
Shrimp, mixed species, raw	1 medium piece	6	0	1	0	0
Snacks, cheese puffs or twists	1 oz.	157	10	2	15	0
Soda, club	12 fl.oz.	0	0	0	0	0
Soda, cream	12 fl.oz.	252	0	0	66	0
Soda, diet cola	12 fl.oz.	0	0	0	0	0
Soda, ginger ale	12 fl.oz.	166	0	0	43	0
Soda, lemon-lime	12 fl.oz.	196	0	0	51	0
Soda, regular, w/ caffeine	12 fl.oz.	155	0	0	40	0
Soda, regular, w/o caffeine	12 fl.oz.	207	0	0	53	0
Soda, root beer	12 fl.oz.	202	0	0	52	0
Soda, tonic water	12 fl.oz.	166	0	0	43	0
Soup, beef broth	1 cup	29	0	5	2	0
Soup, beef stroganoff	1 cup	235	11	12	22	1
Soup, beef vegetable	1 cup	82	2	3	13	1
Soup, chicken broth	1 cup	39	1	5	1	0
Soup, chicken noodle	1 cup	75	2	4	9	1
Soup, chicken vegetable	1 cup	75	3	4	9	1
Soup, chicken w/ dumplings	1 cup	96	6	6	6	1
Soup, clam chowder	1 cup	95	3	5	12	2
Soup, cream of chicken	1 cup	117	7	3	9	0

Nutrition values for fat, protein (Prtn), carbohydrates (Cbs), and fiber (Fbr) are listed in grams per serving. Serving sizes and values are approximate.

FOOD ITEM	Serving Size	Cal	Fat	Prtn	Cbs	Fbr
S (cont.)						
Soup, cream of mushroom	1 cup	129	9	2	9	1
Soup, cream of potato	1 cup	149	6	6	17	1
Soup, minestrone	1 cup	82	3	4	11	1
Soup, split-pea w/ham	1 cup	190	4	10	28	2
Soup, tomato	1 cup	161	6	6	22	3
Soup, vegetarian	1 cup	72	2	2	12	1
Sour cream	1 tbsp	26	2.5	0	1	0
Sour cream, fat free	1 tbsp	9	0	0	2	0
Sour cream, reduced fat	1 tbsp	22	2	1	1	0
Soy milk	1 cup	127	5	11	12	3
Soy protein isolate	1 oz.	96	1	23	2	2
Soybeans, green, cooked	1 cup	254	12	22	12	7
Soybeans, nuts, roasted	1/4 cup	194	9	17	14	3
Soyburger	1 patty	125	4	13	9	3
Spaghetti, cooked	1 cup	197	1	7	40	2
Spaghetti, spinach, cooked	1 cup	182	1	6	37	2
Spaghetti, whole-wheat, cooked	1 cup	174	1	7	37	6
Spinach	1 cup	7	0	1	1	1
Squab, boneless, raw	1 squab	585	47	37	0	0
Squab, skinless, raw	1 squab	239	13	29	0	0
Squash, summer	1 cup, sliced	18	0	1	4	1
Squash, winter	1 cup, cubed	39	0	1	10	2
Squid, mixed species, raw	1 oz.	26	0	4	1	0
Stock, beef	1 cup	31	0	5	3	0
Stock, chicken	1 cup	86	3	6	9	0
Stock, fish	1 cup	40	2	5	0	0
Strawberries	1 cup	49	1	1	12	3
Succotash	1 piece	0	0	0	0	0
Sugar, brown	1 tsp	12	0	0	3	0
Sugar, granulated	1 tsp	16	0	0	4	0
Sugar, maple	1 tsp	11	0	0	3	0
Sugar, powdered	1 tsp	10	0	0	3	0
Sunflower seeds	1 tbsp	45	10	4	2	5
Sweet potato	1 cup, cubed	114	0	2	27	4
Syrup, chocolate	1 tbsp	67	2	1	12	1
Syrup, dark corn	1 tbsp	57	0	0	16	0
Syrup, grenadine	1 tbsp	53	0	0	13	0
Syrup, light corn	1 tbsp	59	0	0	16	0
Syrup, maple	1 tbsp	52	0	0	13	0
Syrup, pancake	1 tbsp	47	0	0	12	0

Nutrition values for fat, protein (Prtn), carbohydrates (Cbs), and fiber (Fbr)
are listed in grams per serving. Serving sizes and values are approximate.

FOOD ITEM	Serving Size	Cal	Fat	Prtn	Cbs	Fbr
T						
Taco shell, hard	1 shell	55	3	2	6	0
Tangerines	1 large	52	0	1	13	2
Tarragon, dried	1 tsp	2	0	0	0	0
Tea, instant	1 cup	2	0	0	0	0
Thyme	1 tsp	1	0	0	0	0
Thyme, dried	1 tsp	3	0	0	1	0
Tofu, firm	1/2 cup	183	11	20	5	3
Tofu, fried	1 piece	35	3	2	1	1
Tofu, soft	1/2 cup	76	5	8	2	0
Tomato juice, canned, with salt	6 fl.oz.	31	0	1	8	1
Tomato juice, canned, without salt	6 fl.oz.	30	0	1	8	1
Tomato paste, canned	1/2 cup	107	1	6	25	6
Tomato sauce, canned	1 cup	78	1	3	18	4
Tomatoes, canned, crushed	1 cup	82	1	4	19	5
Tomatoes, green	1 cup, chopped	41	0	2	9	2
Tomatoes, orange	1 cup, chopped	25	0	2	5	1
Tomatoes, red	1 cup, chopped	32	0	2	7	2
Tomatoes, sun-dried	1 cup, chopped	139	2	8	30	7
Toppings, butterscotch or caramel	2 tbsp	103	0	1	27	0
Toppings, marshmallow cream	2 tbsp	132	0	0	32	0
Toppings, nuts in syrup	2 tbsp	184	9	2	24	1
Toppings, pineapple	2 tbsp	106	0	0	28	0
Toppings, strawberry	2 tbsp	107	0	0	28	0
Tortilla chips, plain	1 oz.	142	7	2	18	2
Tortilla, corn	1 tortilla	45	1	2	9	3
Tortilla, flour	1 tortilla	160	3	18	28	3
Trail mix	1/4 cup	173	11	5	17	3
Turkey, deli sliced, white meat	1 oz.	30	1	5	1	0
Turkey, back, skinless, boneless, raw	1/2 back	180	5	31	0	0
Turkey, breast, boneless, raw	1/2 breast	541	12	103	0	0
Turkey, breast, skinless, boneless, raw	1/2 breast	433	3	96	0	0
Turkey, dark meat, boneless, raw	1/2 turkey	686	26	107	0	0
Turkey, dark meat, skinless, boneless, raw	1/2 turkey	532	13	98	0	0
Turkey, leg, boneless, raw	1 leg	412	13	70	0	0
Turkey, leg, skinless, boneless, raw	1 leg	355	8	67	0	0
Turkey, wing, boneless, raw	1 wing	204	10	27	0	0
Turkey, wing, skinless, boneless, raw	1 wing	95	1	20	0	0
Turkey, young hen, back, boneless, raw	1/2 back	650	48	52	0	0
Turkey, young hen, breast, boneless, raw	1/2 breast	1460	73	189	0	0
Turkey, young hen, dark meat, boneless, raw	1/2 turkey	1056	40	163	0	0

Nutrition values for fat, protein (Prtn), carbohydrates (Cbs), and fiber (Fbr) are listed in grams per serving. Serving sizes and values are approximate.

NUTRITION FACTS

FOOD ITEM	Serving Size	Cal	Fat	Prtn	Cbs	Fbr
T (cont.)						
Turkey, young hen, leg, boneless, raw	1 leg	991	49	128	0	0
Turkey, young hen, wing, boneless, raw	1 wing	470	31	45	0	0
Turkey, young tom, back, boneless, raw	1/2 back	938	58	97	0	0
Turkey, young tom, breast, boneless, raw	1/2 breast	2701	113	393	0	0
Turkey, young tom, dark meat, boneless, raw	1/2 turkey	1884	63	307	0	0
Turkey, young tom, leg, boneless, raw	1 leg	1740	78	241	0	0
Turkey, young tom, wing, boneless, raw	1 wing	654	39	71	0	0
Turnip greens	1 cup, chopped	18	0	1	4	2
Turnips	1 cup, cubed	36	0	1	8	2
V						
Vanilla extract	1 tbsp	37	0	0	2	0
Veal, breast, raw	1 oz.	59	4	5	0	0
Veal, cubed, raw	1 oz.	31	1	6	0	0
Veal, ground, raw	1 oz.	41	2	6	0	0
Veal, leg, raw	1 oz.	33	1	6	0	0
Veal, loin, raw	1 oz.	46	3	5	0	0
Veal, rib, raw	1 oz.	46	3	5	0	0
Veal, shank, raw	1 oz.	32	1	5	0	0
Veal, shoulder, arm, raw	1 oz.	37	2	6	0	0
Veal, shoulder, blade, raw	1 oz.	37	2	6	0	0
Veal, shoulder, whole, raw	1 oz.	37	2	6	0	0
Veal, sirloin, raw	1 oz.	43	2	5	0	0
Vegetable juice	8 fl.oz.	50	0	2	12	2
Vinegar	1 tbsp	2	0	0	1	0
W						
Waffles, plain	1 waffle	218	11	6	25	0
Walnuts	1 oz. (14 halves)	185	19	4	4	2
Wasabi root	1 cup, sliced	142	1	6	31	10
Water chestnuts, Chinese	1/2 cup, sliced	60	0	1	15	2
Watercress	1 cup, chopped	4	0	1	0	0
Watermelon	1 cup, diced	46	0	1	12	1
Wheat bran	1 cup	125	3	9	37	25
Wheat flour, whole grain	1 cup	407	2	16	87	15
Wheat germ	1 cup	414	11	27	60	15
Whipped cream	1 cup	154	13	2	8	0
Wine, cooking	1 tsp	2	0	0	0	0
Wine, red	3-1/2 oz. glass	74	0	0	2	0
Wine, rose	3-1/2 oz. glass	73	0	0	1	0

Nutrition values for fat, protein (Prtn), carbohydrates (Cbs), and fiber (Fbr) are listed in grams per serving. Serving sizes and values are approximate.

NUTRITION FACTS

FOOD ITEM	Serving Size	Cal	Fat	Prtn	Cbs	Fbr
W (cont.)						
Wine, white	3-1/2 oz. glass	70	0	0	1	0
Y						
Yam	1 cup, cubed	177	0	2	42	6
Yeast, active, dry	1 tsp	12	0	2	2	1
Yogurt, fruit, low fat	8 oz. container	118	0	6	24	0
Yogurt, fruit, whole milk	8 oz. container	250	6	9	38	0
Yogurt, plain, lowfat	8 oz. container	110	4	8	7	0
Yogurt, plain, whole milk	8 oz. container	138	7	12	11	0
Z						
Zucchini	1 medium	45	0	2	10	1

Nutrition values for fat, protein (Prtn), carbohydrates (Cbs), and fiber (Fbr) are listed in grams per serving. Serving sizes and values are approximate.

NUTRITION FACTS

Notes:

Tell Us Your Weight-Loss Success Story!

We love hearing when our readers lose 10 pounds or 2 clothing sizes in just two weeks!

Please tell us your story, your initial weight and measurements, your expectations for this diet and fitness program, etc. Tell us what you liked or didn't like about this book, and what you found useful or wished we had included. Tell us how difficult or how easy it was for you to stick to your diet or maintain the exercise program. Now, tell us how you feel with your new slimmer and healthier body. Share your best advice for others who are struggling with their weight.

Please include the following information:

- Your name:
- Phone number:
- E-mail:
- Your story!
- Before and After photos, if possible

Please email this information to info@WSPublishingGroup.com or send a letter to WS Publishing Group, 7290 Navajo Road, Suite 207; San Diego, CA 92119.